Cancer Screening in the Developing World

Geisel Series in Global Health and Medicine

SERIES EDITORS

Lisa V. Adams, MD, associate professor of medicine and associate dean for global health at Geisel School of Medicine at Dartmouth

John R. Butterly, MD, professor of medicine at Geisel School of Medicine at Dartmouth and the Dartmouth Institute of Health Policy and Clinical Practice

This series, sponsored by Dartmouth College Press, draws on the scholarly and practical expertise of a diverse group of health care practitioners and public health professionals engaged in combatting a wide range of challenging health issues faced by low-income countries around the globe. Books in the series vary: they may focus on a geographical area, such as Central America; a specific topic, such as surgery; or a particular set of health issues in their environmental and political contexts. All books in the series should speak to medical students, health care and public health professionals, and anyone interested in engaging in global health work or learning more about the issues and problems facing our global society.

For a complete list of books that are available in the series, visit www.upne.com

Madelon L. Finkel, editor, *Cancer Screening in the Developing World: Case Studies and Strategies from the Field*

Kathleen Allden and Nancy Murakami, editors, *Trauma and Recovery on War's Border: A Guide for Global Health Workers*

Lisa V. Adams and John R. Butterly, *Diseases of Poverty: Epidemiology, Infectious Diseases, and Modern Plagues*

Margo J. Krasnoff, editor, *Building Partnerships in the Americas: A Guide for Global Health Workers*

Anji E. Wall, *Ethics for International Medicine: A Practical Guide for Aid Workers in Developing Countries*

Kate Tulenko, *Insourced: How Importing Jobs Impacts the Healthcare Crisis Here and Abroad*

Laurel A. Spielberg and Lisa V. Adams, editors, *Africa: A Practical Guide for Global Health Workers*

John R. Butterly and Jack Shepherd, *Hunger: The Biology and Politics of Starvation*

CANCER SCREENING IN THE DEVELOPING WORLD

Edited by Madelon L. Finkel, PhD

Dartmouth College Press | Hanover, New Hampshire

Dartmouth College Press
An imprint of University Press of New England
www.upne.com
© 2018 Trustees of Dartmouth College
All rights reserved
Manufactured in the United States of America
Designed by April Leidig
Typeset in Minion by Copperline Book Services, Inc.

For permission to reproduce any of the material in this book, contact
Permissions, University Press of New England, One Court Street,
Suite 250, Lebanon NH 03766; or visit www.upne.com

Library of Congress Cataloging-in-Publication Data
Names: Finkel, Madelon Lubin, 1949– editor.
Title: Cancer screening in the developing world : case studies and
    strategies from the field / edited by Madelon L. Finkel.
Description: Hanover, New Hampshire : Dartmouth College
    Press, [2018] | Series: Geisel series in global health and medicine |
    Includes bibliographical references and index.
Identifiers: LCCN 2017048806 (print) | LCCN 2017049784 (ebook) |
    ISBN 9781512602524 (epub, mobi, & pdf) | ISBN 9781512602500
    (hbk. : alk. paper) | ISBN 9781512602517 (pbk. : alk. paper) |
    ISBN 9781512602524 (ebook)
Subjects: | MESH: Early Detection of Cancer | Developing Countries |
    Organizational Case Studies
Classification: LCC RA645.C3 (ebook) | LCC RA645.C3 (print) | NLM QZ 241 |
    DDC 362.19699/40091724—dc23
LC record available at https://lccn.loc.gov/2017048806

5 4 3 2 1

*To the dedicated health care workers
who do so much to help better the lives
of so many in the developing world*

Contents

David Weller

Foreword

The unequal burden of cancer around the world is a major international issue of concern, which makes this book important and timely. Cancer is one of the leading causes of death and disability in low- and middle-income countries (LMICs), where over half of new cancer cases and 65 percent of cancer deaths occur. (1) The underlying causes of the rising cancer incidence and mortality in LMICs include an increase in life expectancy, primarily due to a decrease in the incidence of many infectious diseases that had been leading causes of death. The adoption of Western habits, especially smoking, a sedentary lifestyle, and changes in diet, has also helped fuel the dramatic increase in chronic diseases in LMICs, especially heart disease and cancer. (2) Furthermore, LMICs are affected disproportionately by infectious agents associated with many cancers, such as human papillomavirus (HPV), H. pylori, and hepatitis B. (3) Conversely, Western countries have seen significant improvements in cancer outcomes over the last several decades brought about by reduction in risk factors, but perhaps more important by screening and early diagnosis of cancers followed by effective treatment regimes. (4)

As highlighted by several authors in this book, too many areas of the world are currently without access to any significant early diagnosis and cancer screening programs, which means that cancers typically present at a late stage, resulting in poor survival and significant morbidity. Many LMICs lack the health infrastructure, trained providers, diagnostic and treatment facilities, and affordable therapeutics to reduce the gap between high- and low-income countries. For example, only 19 percent of women are screened for cervical cancer in LMICs, compared to over 60 percent in developed countries. (1)

Many organizations, such as the World Health Organization (WHO), the World Bank, philanthropic foundations (such as the Bill and Melinda Gates Foundation), and the Global Taskforce on Expanded Access to Cancer Control, provide guidance on developing prevention and treatment strategies in LMICs. Such resources provide practical implementation and evaluation strategies. (5,6) However, whichever model is adopted, it is important for the sponsor, whether a government or a nonprofit organization, to address the basic principles of screening (see chapter 2), including community acceptance and economic sustainability.

This book highlights the successes as well as the challenges faced by sponsors of cancer screening programs in various parts of the developing world. The authors describe program strategies and the challenges of developing an effective infrastructure needed for a successful population-based screening program. Take, for example, oral cavity cancer screening. There is evidence to support the use of simple, low-cost screening techniques in poor, rural communities. (7) Yet to date in poor, rural communities where the need is great, there are few oral cavity cancer screening programs that put this evidence into practice. Studies consistently show low levels of awareness of oral cavity cancer among the population. Known carcinogenic agents (including betel nut, chewing tobacco, cigarettes, and alcohol) are available with little restriction in many parts of the world where oral cavity cancer is highly prevalent. Routine oral inspection is rarely done. The end result is a high incidence of late-stage oral cavity cancer and high mortality.

The examples of LMIC cancer screening programs presented in the chapters that follow focus on those cancers than can be screened for in low-tech settings (such as cervical and oral cancers). Many cancers (including breast, colon, and prostate) are routinely screened for in the developed world but not in the developing world because of a lack of facilities and trained personnel. It is not feasible (logistically or financially) to screen for these cancers in LMICs, especially in rural areas. Sadly, we are a long way from providing well-resourced cancer screening programs in these parts of the world.

The cases presented in the chapters illustrate that there is no "right way" to go about designing and implementing cancer screening programs. What may work well in one location may not work elsewhere. There are many factors that must be taken into account in designing a population-based cancer screening program; one size does not fit all. That being said, LMICs face similar challenges to designing and administering a cancer screening program, as reported by each of the authors. The paucity of trained provid- ers (physician and nonphysician), issues in educating the target population about the importance of cancer screening, designing a plan to treat those who test positive at screening, and finding sufficient funding are a few of the challenges discussed in these chapters. Each program described here designed a plan that would work best in its setting.

Many of the authors discuss challenges in providing treatment for those with positive tests. Rigorous follow-up of screening participants (partic- ularly those who test positive) is essential; there is little point in screen- ing if no action is taken following a positive test, nor is failure to act ethi- cal. As many of the authors explain, there are often significant economic, cultural, and social barriers to participation beyond the test itself. LMICs typically lack the appropriate information infrastructure to support the well-coordinated, population-based screening programs found in many Western countries. A number of strategies are being explored to address this challenge in LMICs, including the use of mobile phone technology, or "mHealth." Even in low resource areas of the world, there is a high level of mobile phone usage, which offers the prospect of adopting mHealth ap- proaches to recruitment, education, and follow-up for patients involved in cancer screening programs. (8)

How, then, can we best address the growing international disparities in cancer outcomes between high-income and low-income countries? Without doubt there is a need to close the gap and reduce the impact of poor cancer outcomes on human suffering in LMICs. Screening and early detection must be part of the solution. Yet there is an ethical dilemma in initiating screen- ing in settings where diagnostic and treatment facilities are inadequate or where the cost of treatment would prove to be prohibitive to those in need of care. If one cannot treat those who test positive, can one ethically initiate a screening program?

Clearly new, creative approaches are necessary if we are to make any significant inroads in reducing the imbalance. Indeed, the proliferation of low-cost, "low-tech" methods to screen for cervical cancer relying on visual inspection with a "screen and treat" approach illustrates the potential for adapting screening strategies to low-resource settings. But to be truly effec- tive in reducing or eliminating cervical cancer, which is easily prevented, it is the opinion of many working in this area that screening alone is not suffi- cient. That is, many have called for the immunization of preadolescent girls and boys with the HPV vaccine in addition to screening women between thirty-five and fifty-five years of age. Such actions would do much to reduce the incidence of cervical cancer in later life.

Another important component of the information infrastructure necessary for successful screening is the development of cancer registries, ideally with population-wide coverage. Without information on incidence, prevalence, and mortality of cancer, it is very difficult to establish an effective national cancer prevention and cancer control initiative. Efforts are under way to build and develop registries in many LMICS. (9)

Dr. Finkel and her colleagues are to be commended for producing an authoritative, timely overview that addresses many of the problems at the heart of poor cancer outcomes in LMICS. Each author stresses the importance of concerted international effort to improve screening activities in poor and developing countries. Key actions include investment in universal high-quality primary care to reduce risk factors, enhance early detection, and facilitate treatment. These efforts need to occur alongside programs to promote healthy behavior. Evidence shows that even a modest investment can lead to significant lifestyle-related improvements and closer engagement with preventive activities. (10)

The authors highlight the need for more research on implementation of cancer screening in LMICS by addressing the many individual, cultural, economic, and societal barriers that keep screening rates low. The cases presented poignantly illustrate what can be done to help save lives and what challenges remain.

References

1. Akinyemiju TF. Socio-economic and health access determinants of breast and cervical cancer screening in low-income countries: analysis of the World Health Survey. PloS One 2012;7(11):e48834.

2. Knaul FM, Atun R, Farmer P, Frenk J. Seizing the opportunity to close the cancer divide. Lancet 2013;381(9885):2238.

3. Simard EP, Jemal A. Commentary: infection-related cancers in low-and middle-income countries: challenges and opportunities. Int J Epidemiol 2013;42(1):228–9.

4. De Angelis R, Sant M, Coleman MP, et al. Cancer survival in Europe 1999–2007 by country and age: results of EUROCARE-5—a population-based study. Lancet Oncol 2013 [cited 2013 Dec 5]. Available from: http://dx.doi.org/10.1016/S1470-2045 (13)70546-1.

5. Farmer P, Freno J, Knaul FM, et al. Expansion of cancer care and control in countries of low and middle income: a call to action. Lancet 2010;376(9747):1186–93.

6. Jeronimo J, Castle PE, Temin S, et al. Secondary prevention of cervical cancer:

ASCO resource-stratified clinical practice guideline. J Glob Oncol 2016; Oct 12: JGO006577.

7. Sankaranarayanan R, Ramadas K, Thomas G, et al. Trivandrum oral cancer screening study group: effect of screening on oral cancer mortality in Kerala, India: a cluster-randomised controlled trial. Lancet 2005;365(9475):1927–33.

8. Holeman I, Evans J, Kane D, et al. Mobile health for cancer in low to middle income countries: priorities for research and development. Eur J Cancer Care 2014;23(6):750–6.

9. Bray F, Znaor A, Cueva P et al. Planning and developing population-based cancer registration in low- and middle-income settings. Lyon, France: International Agency for Research on Cancer; 2014/2015. IARC Technical Publication No. 43 [cited 2017 Jan 25]. Available from: http://www.iarc.fr/en/publications/pdfs-online /treport-pub/treport-pub43/.

10. Ranganathan M, Lagarde M. Promoting healthy behaviours and improving health outcomes in low and middle income countries: a review of the impact of conditional cash transfer programmes. Prev Med 2012;55:S95–10.

Cancer Screening in the Developing World

Chapter 1

Madelon L. Finkel

Global Burden of Disease

A Short Overview

T he world has been undergoing a major shift over the past few decades in the incidence and prevalence of diseases as well as in the leading causes of death. Diseases that once were highly prevalent (and usually deadly) are no longer so, and diseases that were not prevalent in the past are now at the top of the list. Whereas for many decades infectious disease morbidity and mortality was the prime focus of concern, especially in the developing world, today chronic, non-communicable diseases (NCDs) are.

Quantifying "the global burden of disease" is challenging at best. The World Health Organization (WHO) arrived at a broad consensus definition of global burden of disease (GBD) in the mid-1990s to reflect the collective disease burden produced by all diseases around the world. (1) In an effort to define the concept more specifically, the WHO uses the disability-adjusted life year (DALY) to measure "burden of disease." The DALY was developed in the 1990s as a way of comparing overall health and life expectancy among different countries. Essentially, it is a measure of overall disease burden expressed as the number of years lost due to ill-health, disability, or early death, and years of life lost due to time lived in states of less than full health or years of healthy life lost due to disability. However, obtaining accurate, valid statistics from countries is difficult, and in some cases almost impossible. Because so many factors have an impact on disease, political, social, and economic determinants of health must be taken into account, and these factors vary widely not only among countries, but also within them.

Almost all of the data presented in this chapter are abstracted from The Global Burden of Disease Study 2015 (GBD 2015), a comprehensive, worldwide observational epidemiological study that assesses mortality and disability from major diseases, injuries, and risk factors. The study relies on more than 80,000 data sources, drawing from the world's largest global health database and focusing on 125 countries and 3 territories. Almost 2,000 collaborators contributed to the reports. (2)

The GBD studies examine trends from 1990 to the present and make comparisons across populations. The GBD project, initially sponsored by the World Bank and conducted by the WHO, presents a historical, comprehensive look at changing morbidity and mortality patterns worldwide from 1990 to 2015. The GBD 2015 is the most recent in the series. The studies provide a comprehensive, global estimate of death and disease by age, sex, and country. Based on the GBD statistics, it is apparent that the world is experiencing an "epidemiological/demographic transition." There has been a noticeable shift in global deaths and disability in recent decades; overall, life expectancy is rising in most parts of the world. This chapter presents a broad overview of the GBD, including disease prevalence, incidence, and mortality in the developed and developing world.

The Demographic Transition and Its Effects on Mortality and Life Expectancy

Over the past couple of centuries the world experienced a demographic transition characterized by a transition from high birth and death rates to lower birth and death rates. The Demographic Transition Model describes a process that began in Europe in the early 1800s, characterized by decreases in mortality followed, usually after a time lag, by decreases in fertility. (3) Under this model, initially both birth and death rates are high and natural population growth is low. As mortality begins to fall, fertility still remains high. As fertility begins to fall, there is a reduction in birthrates, eventually resulting in a reduction in the rate of population growth.

Somewhat simplistically, there is a transition from high birth and death rates to lower birth and death rates primarily because of advances in medicine, hygiene, public health, and economics. Reductions in mortality and birthrates reduce population growth, accelerate human capital formation, and increase income per capita. Demographers have shown a strong link between number of live births, infant mortality, and women's education. (4) Further, reductions in the birthrate are closely linked to higher labor force participation rates among women. (5) The end result is that life expectancy increases and premature death, notably infant and child mortality, decreases.

Worldwide, people are living much longer today than they were even two decades ago. Overall, life expectancy was 71.4 years in 2015, with an average life expectancy for women of 73.8 years and 69.1 years for men. From 2000 to 2015 global average life expectancy increased by 5 years, primarily as a result of improvements in child survival and expanded access to antiretrovirals for treatment of HIV. (6) Of course these estimates must be interpreted with caution, especially given recent geopolitical events such as forced migration, wars, famine, and drought that jeopardize gains made in life expectancy around the world.

Reflecting the trend in increased life expectancy, country age pyramids in the twenty-first century look quite different from those in the twentieth century. Whereas most places in the developed world have an aging population (the United States, Europe, and Australia in particular), countries in the developing world have a surging younger population *as well as* an aging population. Although gains in life expectancy have been shown for almost all countries, there is substantial variation within and across countries. Overall, Monaco leads the list of countries with the highest life expectancy, 89.5 years, with Japan second, at 85 years. In stark contrast, Chad posts the lowest life expectancy (49.8 years). (7) Within countries there are substantial differences in life expectancy. For example, in 2014 in the United States, life expectancy for Caucasians was 79.1 years, compared to 75.5 years for African Americans and 82.9 years for Hispanics. There are also substantial variations by gender, and Hispanic women and men have the highest life expectancy among ethnic groups in the United States. (8)

Changing Patterns in Mortality

The GBD 2015 shows global changes in deaths in adults and children. While the number of deaths and age-standardized death rates for communicable diseases fell between 1990 and 2015, there was an increase in age-standardized death rates for diabetes, atrial fibrillation and flutter, some cancers (such as pancreatic), drug use disorders, cirrhosis, and chronic kidney disease. In particular, drug use disorders and chronic kidney disease account for the largest percent increase in premature deaths.

Infectious diseases remain among the top five causes of death in the developing world and the top ten causes of death in the developed world.

Lower respiratory infection (used as a synonym for pneumonia in the GBD 2015 study) ranks number one in cause of death in low-income countries (compared to number seven in high-income countries). HIV/AIDS, despite tremendous progress made in treatment and survival, ranks number two in low-income countries but is not in the top ten causes of death in high-income countries. Almost a decade after HIV/AIDS peaked globally, this disease still substantially contributes to premature death. It continues to ravage sub-Saharan Africa and has had a profound impact on life expectancy in that region. Diarrheal disease is the third leading cause of death in low-income countries but is not in the top ten causes of death in high-income countries.

Trends in age-sex-specific, all-cause, and cause-specific mortality show that since 1990 there have been substantial shifts in disease mortality worldwide. However, the data clearly show variations by age, sex, and country, including differences within countries. (9) In high-income countries, people predominantly die of chronic disease: cardiovascular disease, cancer, dementia, chronic obstructive lung disease, and diabetes. Lower respiratory tract infection is the only infectious disease in the top ten causes of death in these countries. Conversely, in low-income countries, people predominantly die of infectious diseases: lower respiratory infection, HIV/AIDS, diarrheal disease, malaria, and tuberculosis. Complications of childbirth due to prematurity, birth asphyxia, and birth trauma are also among the leading causes of death in low-income countries, especially in the rural, poor areas of the world.

Ninety-nine percent of all maternal deaths occur in developing countries (especially in much of sub-Saharan Africa), and the rate is higher among women living in rural areas and poorer communities. (10) Since the 1980s there has been a global effort to reduce maternal mortality; the United Nations Millennium Development Goal 5 specifically established a goal of a 75 percent reduction in the maternal mortality rate. For many reasons this goal was not realized despite major advances in obstetrical care. Rather than setting broad-based targets, it is probably more prudent to set regional goals and push for effecting change in those areas of the world that are lagging behind. The Millennium Development Goals (MDGs) are eight specific goals, including measurable targets, designed to improve the lives of the world's poorest people. To meet these goals and eradicate poverty, leaders of 189 countries signed the declaration at the United Nations Millennium Summit in 2000.

While there has been substantial global progress made in reducing child deaths since 1990, in 2015 seventy-nine countries had an under-five mortality rate above 25 deaths per 1,000 live births. Overall, children in sub-Saharan Africa are more likely to die before age five than children in other parts of the world. The leading causes of death in this group continue to be diarrheal disease, lower respiratory tract infections, neonatal disorders, and malaria. The majority of these causes of death could be prevented or treated successfully if affordable interventions were available. Diarrhea due to rotavorius and measles, for example, kill more than 1 million children under age five every year, even though there are effective vaccines against those diseases. (11) That being said, there are wide gaps in child mortality across subgroups and areas within countries.

Changes in lifestyle, behavior, and diet, now rapidly spreading in the developing world, contribute substantially to the shift in causes of death. For example, the rising global epidemic of obesity has directly contributed to the huge increase in the incidence of cardiovascular disease and diabetes in both the developed and developing worlds. Despite global antismoking campaigns and local and state laws prohibiting smoking in indoor public spaces, the WHO estimates that tobacco smoking is responsible for approximately 10 percent of all deaths globally. (12) Nearly 80 percent of the world's 1 billion smokers live in low- and middle-income countries.

The proportion of deaths due to NCDS is projected to rise from 59 percent in 2002 to 69 percent in 2030. (13) The current leading cause-specific deaths are cardiovascular disease (ischemic heart disease and stroke), respiratory disease (including pneumonia and chronic obstructive pulmonary disease [COPD]), and diabetes. Ischemic heart disease contributes 13.2 percent to total global deaths. Stroke, the second leading cause of death worldwide, contributes 11.9 percent to total deaths. Both conditions are highly prevalent in the developed and the developing worlds, although there are significant geographical differences in stroke burden among regions and countries. While age-standardized rates of stroke mortality have decreased worldwide, the absolute number of individuals who have strokes is increasing. (14)

Injuries continue to be an important cause of morbidity and mortality in the developed and developing worlds, accounting for 10.1 percent of the global burden of disease in 2015. Approximately 973 million people sustained injuries that warranted some type of health care, and almost 5 million died from their injuries. The GBD 2015 study clearly showed that globally, vehicular injury among all age groups remains the ninth leading cause of death, while it is the leading cause of death among those between fifteen and twenty-nine years old. Road traffic injuries alone contributed to the death of 5 million people each year, or 3,400 lives each day. Road highway deaths are higher in low-income countries than in middle-income or high-income countries. By continent, road traffic fatalities are the highest in Africa (26.6 per 100,000 people) and the lowest in Europe (9.3 per 100,000 people). (14)

In summary, the data clearly indicate a shift in disease mortality over time. By 2015 the leading causes of death were NCDs that are lifestyle related; these diseases accounted for half of all deaths globally. The evidence shows that over the past few decades, countries experiencing economic development (such as Brazil, Russia, India, and China) have seen more rapid changes in lifestyle, behavior, and diet, which subsequently have had a negative impact on health status and mortality. Modernization can be a double-edged sword.

Changing Patterns of Morbidity

Although people are living longer, most are living with chronic conditions and increased disability, requiring long-term treatment, medication, and monitoring. As economic prosperity creates a growing middle class, it brings with it not only personal wealth but also a dramatic shift in lifestyle, especially including changes in traditional diet. India and China, in particular, are prime examples of this global transition of disease. This new middle class has embraced a "Western" lifestyle characterized by Western habits such as high-fat diets, reduced physical activity, increased alcohol consumption, and tobacco smoking. Not surprisingly, there has been a surge in the incidence and prevalence of "Western" diseases such as cardiovascular disease, hypertension, cancer, and especially diabetes mellitus, primarily due to obesity and being overweight. People are living longer, but they are living longer with chronic diseases that require daily medication and careful monitoring.

The leading causes of morbidity in 2015 illustrate a shift from communicable diseases to lifestyle-related conditions. At the top of the list is ischemic heart disease; smoking; the consumption of high-cholesterol, high-fat foods; stress; high blood pressure; diabetes; abdominal obesity; lack of exercise; and excessive alcohol consumption all contribute to the development of ischemic heart disease. COPD and lower respiratory infections are prevalent around the world. COPD is caused primarily by tobacco smoking and air pollution (in the home and in the workplace). Lower respiratory infections, inclusive of pneumonia, influenza, bronchitis, and bronchiolitis, are aggravated by air pollution (indoor and outdoor), tobacco smoke, and smoke from burning solid fuel such as firewood. Whereas COPD is more prevalent among older people, lower respiratory infections are common among children, especially those younger than age five who live in developing countries. (15)

While the numbers of malnourished children worldwide have been reduced (with the exception of sub-Saharan Africa, which continues to present a myriad of challenges for a variety of geographic, medical, and economic reasons), poor diets and physical inactivity are contributing to rising rates of obesity, hypertension, and especially diabetes. In particular, the prevalence of diabetes worldwide is huge and growing. An estimated 422 million people worldwide have diabetes, and this number is projected to increase substantially over time. In 1990 diabetes was tenth on the list of leading diseases; in 2015, it ranked seventh. Diabetes was responsible for an estimated 1.5 million deaths in 2012. (16)

Diabetes and its complications contribute to substantial economic losses for individuals and their families as well as society in general. Disability resulting from diabetes has grown substantially since 1990, with particularly large increases among people fifteen to sixty-nine years old. (17) Being overweight or obese, combined with physical inactivity, is responsible for a substantial proportion of the global diabetes burden.

The increase in obesity and being overweight worldwide is striking and is now a major global public health challenge. The worldwide prevalence of obesity more than doubled between 1980 and 2014. Globally, the proportion of adults with a body mass index (BMI) of 25 or greater increased between 1980 and 2015 from almost 29 percent to almost 37 percent in males and from almost 30 percent to 38 percent in women. These increases were found in both the developed and developing worlds. Moreover, there have been substantial increases in the proportion of obese and overweight children and adolescents, especially in the developed world. The proportion of overweight and obese children and adolescents in the developing world is also rapidly increasing. (18)

Globally, an estimated 1 billion people have high blood pressure, and two-thirds of them live in developing countries. This "silent disease" is a major contributor to the global burden of disease and to global mortality, and it is estimated to cause half of all deaths from stroke and heart disease. (19)

Since the launch of the DALY in 1993, the burden of disease concept has become more widely adopted by countries and health development agencies. The global burden of disability (including such conditions as lower back pain, depressive disorder, age-related and other hearing loss, and neck pain) is increasing as the population ages. That being said, the leading causes of disability vary considerably with age: among children younger than five years old, iron-deficiency anemia ranks as the top cause, followed by skin diseases, protein-energy malnutrition, and diarrhea. Among middle-aged adults, musculoskeletal disorders and mental health disorders (especially depression) are prevalent. The burden of mental and substance use disorders increased by 37.6 percent between 1990 and 2010, primarily due to population growth and aging. Overall, however, depression is considered to be the most disabling disorder worldwide, based on years lived with disability (YLD), and the fourth leading cause of overall disease burden measured in DALYs. (20) Among those age sixty-five and older, sense organ disorders were the top-ranked cause of disability, followed by musculoskeletal disorders. There has also been an increase in the prevalence of Alzheimer's and other dementias among the elderly, especially in the developed countries. (20)

The GBD 2015 study also showed that since 1990 there has been a decrease in the rate of DALYs among the major causes of injury (such as acts of violence against others or oneself, road traffic crashes, burns, drowning, falls, and poisonings); however, the patterns vary widely by cause, age, sex, region, and time. (20)

In summary, modern medicine and advances in public health have done much to increase life expectancy for millions who otherwise would have died at a younger age because of disease. The data are clear that NCDs have surpassed communicable diseases as leading causes of morbidity and mortality not only in the developed world, but also in much of the developing world. Globally, three conditions accounted for almost one-third of all deaths in 2015: ischemic heart disease, stroke, and COPD. (21) This is not to say that we have eliminated the burden of infectious disease; quite the contrary. The 2015 Ebola and 2016 Zika virus outbreaks are clear illustrations that infectious diseases can, and do, cause havoc worldwide. Tuberculosis, malaria, cholera, and HIV/AIDS stubbornly remain major causes of morbidity and mortality in many parts of the world. However, countries have made great strides in reducing mortality from diseases such as measles and polio.

While the developed world transitioned from communicable to non-communicable diseases many years ago, most developing countries are now experiencing and coping with a dual burden of disease management. This burden challenges the finances and capacities of most health systems. Today, individuals are living longer but with chronic, long-term conditions. These chronic diseases are costly to manage, and many countries do not have the skilled personnel to handle the sheer numbers of individuals requiring short- and long-term care. Many countries also are hard pressed to allocate sufficient funding for the necessary long-term treatment.

Focus on Cancer

According to the WHO, "cancer is the second leading cause of death globally, responsible for 8.8 million deaths in 2015. Globally, nearly 1 in 6 deaths is due to cancer. Of this, approximately 70 percent of deaths from cancer occur in low- and middle-income countries." (22) Late-stage presentation is common in most low-income countries. In 2015 only 35 percent of low-income countries reported having pathology services generally available in the public sector. (22)

Breast cancer is the most common cancer in women in both the developed and less-developed worlds, with an estimated 1.67 million new cancer cases diagnosed in 2012 (25% of all cancers). While breast cancer is the most frequent cause of cancer death in women in less-developed regions (as of 2012, 324,000 deaths, 14.3% of the total), it is now the second cause of cancer death in more developed regions (as of 2012, 198,000 deaths, 15.4%) after lung cancer. (23)

Cervical cancer is the fourth leading cause of death among women worldwide, and the seventh cause of death overall, with an estimated 528,000 new cases in 2012. There were an estimated 266,000 deaths from cervical cancer worldwide in 2012, accounting for 7.5 percent of all female cancer deaths. However, the overwhelming majority of cases occur in the developing world, accounting for almost 12 percent of all female cancers. (24) The tragedy is that cervical cancer can be easily treated if detected at an early stage. Almost all cases of cervical cancer are due to infection by human papillomavirus (HPV), especially HPV 16 and 18. Screening to detect precancerous lesions has been shown to be highly effective in reducing the incidence of late-stage cancer. Chapters 4, 5, 6, and 7 address cervical cancer screening, diagnosis, and treatment in more depth.

Oral cavity cancer is a growth of malignant cells in any part of the oral cavity, which includes the lips, tongue, hard and soft palates, salivary glands, lining of the cheeks, floor of the mouth or under the tongue, gums, and teeth. Oropharyngeal cancers form in tissues of the oropharynx (the part of the throat at the back of the mouth, including the soft palate, the base of the tongue, and the tonsils). The most common site of oral cavity cancer is the lip, followed by the tongue and then other locations. Oral cavity cancers are among the most prevalent cancers worldwide; incidence rates are higher in men than women. (25) These cancers often go undetected; the cancer is usually discovered when the malignant cells have metastasized, most likely to the lymph nodes of the neck. In general, the prognosis for survival is poor. Risk factors include age (although cases are now seen in individuals younger than age forty), tobacco smoking and smokeless tobacco, alcohol consumption, and persistent viral infections such as HPV. Chapter 8 in this book provides a more in-depth discussion of oral cavity cancer screening and diagnosis.

Summary

This chapter has presented a snapshot of the global burden of disease. Much more detailed information can be found in the numerous published studies based on the GBD 2015. Clearly progress has been made in reducing mortality from many diseases since 1990, but the increase in NCDs around the world presents many challenges. In particular, developing countries bear a disproportionate share of the global burden of disease, perhaps because of the paucity of health personnel and facilities, the lack of medications, the lack of funding to provide care, and country-specific politics. Likewise, within countries the burden of disease tends to fall inequitably on the poorer, less-advantaged population.

The significant increase in NCDs worldwide, coupled with the existing burden of communicable diseases (dual burden of disease), poses a challenge to managing the health of the global population. Perhaps leveraging technology is one way to address this problem. Perhaps information technology, coupled with advances in public health and medicine, could prove to be a winning combination in disease management and prevention in the future.

Acknowledgment

This book could not have been written without the assistance of my research staff, Maritza Montalvo and Sejal Shah. Their help in preparing the manuscript is much appreciated.

References

1. World Health Organization. Global burden of disease [cited 2016 Jul 9]. Available from: http://www.who.int/topics/global_burden_of_disease/en/.

2. The Global Burden of Disease Study 2015. Lancet 2016;388(10053): 1447–1850.

3. Grover D. What is the demographic transition model? Population Education; 2014 Oct 13 [cited 2016 Jul 9]. Available from: https://www.populationeducation.org/content/what-demographic-transition-model.

4. Desai S, Alva S. Maternal education and child health: is there a strong causal relationship? Demogr 1998;35:71–81.

5. Guinnane TW. The historical fertility transition: a guide for economists. J Econ Lit 2011; 9(3):589–614.

6. World Health Organization. Life expectancy increased by 5 years since 2000, but health inequalities persist. 2016 May 19 [cited 2016 Jul 9]. Available from: http://www.who.int/mediacentre/news/releases/2016/health-inequalities-persist/en/.

7. Ageing in the twenty-first century: a celebration and a challenge. United Nations Population Fund (UNFPA); 2012 [cited 2016 July 9]. Available from: https://www.unfpa.org/sites/default/files/pub-pdf/Ageing%20report.pdf.

8. Xu J, Murphy SL, Kochanek KD, et al. Deaths: final data for 2013. Natl Vital Stat Rep 2016;64(2) [cited 2016 July 9]. Available from: http://www.cdc.gov/nchs/data/nvsr/nvsr64/nvsr64_02.pdf.

9. Global, regional, and national life expectancy, all-cause mortality, and cause-specific mortality for 249 causes of death, 1980–2015: a systematic analysis for the Global Burden of Disease Study 2015. Lancet 2016;388(10053):1459–1544.

10. Global, regional, and national levels and causes of maternal mortality 1990–2015: a systematic analysis for the Global Burden of Disease Study 2015. Lancet 2016;388(10053): 1775–1812.

11. World Health Organization. Children: reducing mortality. 2016 Sept [cited 2016 Jul 9]. Available from: http://www.who.int/mediacentre/factsheets/fs178/en/.

12. WHO global report on trends in prevalence of tobacco smoking 2015 [cited 2016 Jul 9]. Available from: http://apps.who.int/iris/bitstream/10665/156262/1/9789241564922_eng.pdf.

13. Samet J, Loncar D. Projections of global mortality and burden of disease from 2002 to 2030. PLoS Med 2006;3(11):e442.

14. Global, regional, and national life expectancy, all-cause mortality, and cause-specific mortality for 249 causes of death, 1980–2015: a systematic analysis for the Global Burden of Disease Study 2015. Lancet 2016;388(10053):1459–1544.

15. Institute for Health Metrics and Evaluation. Global burden of disease: massive shifts reshape the health landscape worldwide. 2012 Dec 13 [cited 2016 Jul 9]. Available from: http://www.healthdata.org/news-release/global-burden-disease-massive -shifts-reshape-health-landscape-worldwide.

16. World Health Organization. Report on diabetes. 2016 [cited 2016 Jul 9]. Available from: http://apps.who.int/iris/bitstream/10665/204871/1/9789241565257_eng.pdf.

17. Krug EC. Trends in diabetes: sounding the alarm. Lancet 2016;387(10027): 1485–6, 9.

18. Global, regional and national prevalence of overweight and obesity in children and adults 1980–2013: a systematic review. Lancet 2014;384(9945):766–81.

19. Poulter NR, Prabhakaran D, Caulfiend M. Hypertension. Lancet 2015;386(9995): 801–12.

20. Global, regional, and national incidence, prevalence and years lived with disability for 310 diseases and injuries, 1990–2015: a systematic analysis for the Global Burden of Disease Study 2015. Lancet 2016;388(10053):1545–1602.

21. Global, regional, and national incidence, prevalence, and years lived with disability for 310 diseases and injuries, 1990–2015: a systematic analysis for the Global Burden of Disease Study 2015. Lancet 2016;388(10053):1545–1602.

22. World Health Organization. Cancer fact sheet. 2017 Feb [cited 2017 Apr 24]. Available from: http://www.who.int/mediacentre/factsheets/fs297/en/.

23. Breast cancer estimated incidence, mortality, and prevalence worldwide in 2012 [cited 2016 Jul 9]. Available from: http://globocan.iarc.fr/old/FactSheets/cancers /breast-new.asp.

24. Cervical cancer estimated incidence, mortality, and prevalence worldwide in 2012 [cited 2016 Jul 9]. Available from: http://globocan.iarc.fr/old/FactSheets/cancers /cervix-new.asp.

25. World Health Organization. Global data on incidence of oral cancer [cited 2016 Jul 9]. Available from: http://www.who.int/oral_health/publications/cancer_maps/en/.

Chapter 2

Madelon L. Finkel

The Benefits and Challenges of Population-based Cancer Screening in Low- and Middle-Income Countries

Intellectually and theoretically it is difficult to argue against screening for disease. Who would not want to have a disease detected at an early stage? After all, screening is potentially an excellent way to identify disease in its preclinical, hopefully still curable phase, when early treatment would be beneficial. But as with many things in life, deciding which diseases to screen for and which population groups to screen is not so simple. Not every disease would be appropriate for screening, for many different and important reasons. Should everyone get screened, or should the screening program only target those considered to be at higher risk for developing a particular disease?

Early detection of a disease is admirable, but not alone a sufficient reason to initiate a screening program. Screening must also demonstrate that people would live longer as a result of earlier detection and subsequent treatment. That is, will people who get screened have better survival rates than those who don't get screened? Other important questions need to be addressed, such as the following: How frequently should people be screened for a specific disease? Do the potential benefits outweigh the potential harms of screening? Furthermore, economic, ethical, and clinical issues must be considered before a screening program is implemented. Screening programs are usually costly exercises and do not always deliver the expected benefits in terms of improved health outcomes or longer life expectancy. In some cases, they can do more harm than good.

While many diseases meet the criteria for screening, there are many others that would not qualify as being appropriate or beneficial. This chapter reviews the advantages/benefits of screening programs and discusses their potential harm, with a specific focus on screening for cancer. For potentially fatal conditions such as cancer, a reduction in mortality is one of the most important outcomes to be gained from a screening program. However, consideration must also be given to the quality of life. The mere prolongation of life probably would not adequately justify screening if the quality of the additional life were poor.

Why Screen?

A screening test is designed to identify those who *may* have a disease; they may be healthy with no signs or symptoms or may unknowingly be presymptomatic. That is, a screening test is administered to asymptomatic people, not to those in whom disease has already been diagnosed. Such tests are used to identify individuals who should be referred for further workup so as to arrive at a definitive diagnosis and appropriate treatment. Screening tests are not intended to diagnose disease. They are performed on individuals presumed to be in good health in whom screening will detect disease prior to clinical presentation. And importantly, this implies that the disease should be amenable to treatment when detected at an early stage.

The intention of screening is to diagnose a disease earlier than it would be without screening. In the absence of screening, the disease would be discovered at a later time/later stage, when symptoms appear, and the prognosis would be worse than had the disease been detected earlier. As such, screening can be a valuable public health strategy to help save lives, but only if the potential benefits clearly outweigh the possible harm. Examples are PKU screening in newborns and blood pressure screening in adults.

A "good" screening test should accurately differentiate who has the disease and who does not. That is, the test should be sufficiently sensitive and sufficiently specific. *Sensitivity* is the ability of a test to correctly identify those with the disease (true positive rate), whereas *specificity* is the ability of the test to correctly identify those without the disease (true negative rate). A test with 100 percent sensitivity correctly identifies all patients with the disease. A test with 80 percent sensitivity detects 80 percent of patients with the disease (true positives), but 20 percent with the disease will go undetected (false negatives). A sensitive test helps rule out disease (when the result is negative). Conversely, a test with 100 percent specificity correctly identifies all patients without the disease. A test with 80 percent specificity correctly reports 80 percent of patients without the disease as test negative (true negatives), but 20 percent of the patients without the disease are incorrectly identified as test positive (false positives). A highly specific test means that there are few false positive results.

A test with high sensitivity is more likely to pick up most of those who actually have the disease, which is an important criterion for a screening test. A test with high specificity is unlikely to mislabel people as having the disease if they actually do not. There is always a trade-off between high sensitivity and high specificity. One looks for a balance between the two, which is why determining the cutoff point of a test is so important. In a perfect world, a "perfect test" is never positive in a patient who is disease free and is never negative in a patient who is in fact diseased. In the real world, this is rare. Thus, it is important to understand the rationale for selecting the cutoff point, which will differentiate test positivity from negativity. In general, the higher the sensitivity, the lower the specificity, and vice versa.

Two other characteristics of a screening test are positive predictive value (PPV) and negative predictive value (NPV). *Positive predictive value* is the probability that subjects with a positive screening test truly have the disease. *Negative predictive value* is the probability that subjects with a negative screening test truly do not have the disease. Unlike sensitivity or specificity, PPV and NPV are influenced by the prevalence of disease in the population that is being tested. That is, if we run a screening test in a population among whom the disease prevalence is high, it is more likely that persons who test positive truly have that disease than if the test is performed in a population with low prevalence.

There are instances when a screening test should not be implemented. It could be that there is not a test that is sufficiently sensitive or specific to warrant screening. There are also cases in which the disease would be detected at a late stage even with screening, thus obviating the benefits of screening (such as lung cancer). It could be that the disease is not amenable to screening because no accurate screening tests have been developed (such as ovarian cancer). It could be that the test is too expensive, or that for whatever reason the general public views the test as being not acceptable (perhaps it is too invasive). In short, there are many reasons that screening for a specific disease would not be appropriate. This point is discussed in greater detail in a subsequent section.

Types of Screening

Screening programs come in many different forms. They may be "opportunistic" or "case finding," which refers to an asymptomatic individual actively seeking a screening procedure or a health professional offering a screening test to an asymptomatic individual. Organized screening occurs when there is an organized, population-based program with a structured public health approach.

Population-based screening targets the whole population in a geographic area, such as a program to screen a population for hypertension or diabetes. The screening is available to all regardless of risk status. In contrast, *high-risk screening* programs target only those who are considered to be at higher risk for the disease. For example, one would screen for sickle cell anemia only among an African American cohort because African Americans are at higher risk of developing this disease than other ethnic or racial groups.

Multiphasic community-based screening programs involve the application of two or more screenings at one time instead of conducting separate screening tests for a single disease. Screening for common diseases such as hearing loss, hypertension, and diabetes at a "health fair" is an example of this type. *School-based screening* programs are excellent means to screen schoolchildren for diseases and conditions such as hearing loss, vision, and dental problems.

Screening can also be used to protect a population from exposure to disease (such as tuberculosis [TB]). The primary aim of this type of screening is not to benefit the individual per se, but to protect the local population. Those who test positive for TB should immediately be prescribed medication intended to prevent the spread of this contagious disease. This type of screening relies on case finding, an opportunistic attempt at early detection.

Regardless of the type of screening program, the objectives are the same: to identify those who should be referred for definitive diagnosis of a medical problem and to initiate appropriate treatment. Recommendations for specific screening tests will vary by age, gender, and disease risk factors. As stated previously, not everyone would be a good candidate for a specific screening program. Individuals targeted for screening should be those in whom the prevalence of the disease or the risk of developing the disease is substantial enough to warrant screening. One would not screen for sexually transmitted diseases in a population that is not sexually active, for example. One would not screen for HIV/AIDS in the general population, but screening for this disease in a cohort deemed to be at high risk for this disease would make sense.

What Constitutes a "Good" Screening Test?

An ideal screening test is one for diseases that are considered "serious" if left untreated and are prevalent in the population (including cervical cancer, glaucoma, and diabetes). There is very little point in screening for a disease that few people have (such as gall stones). The screening test must identify a disease that is clinically significant and that, if left untreated, will cause significant morbidity and mortality. In addition, the disease must have a pre-clinical phase, a pre-symptomatic stage in which the disease is detectable. Most important, there must be an acceptable treatment course for those who test positive and have the disease. The test should be reasonably priced, cost-effective, and preferably noninvasive. Screening is very inefficient when the prevalence of the condition is low.

The purpose of screening, however, is not only to detect a condition, but also to enable people to live longer (increased survival). Early detection by itself is probably insufficient to justify a screening program. There has to be evidence that screening contributes to survival, and this implies that there are treatments for the disease that would be available to those who test positive. If the treatment works just as well later in the course of the disease, screening for early detection probably is not warranted. (See table 2.1.)

Guidelines recommending screening are best if based on randomized clinical trials, in which results from a screening program are compared to conventional care or to some gold standard. However, if they are based on evidence from observational studies that show large benefits with a minimal downside, there really isn't a need for a clinical trial. Above all else, before a screening program is implemented, there must be a consensus based on the "best evidence" that the screening program will do more good than harm.

In summary, a "good" screening test should have the following characteristics:

The disease should be an important health problem.
The disease should be sufficiently prevalent in the target population.

Table 2.1. Principles of Early Disease Detection

Condition

The condition should be an important health problem.

There should be a recognizable latent or early symptomatic stage.

The natural history of the condition, including development from latent to declared disease, should be adequately understood.

Test

There should be a suitable test or examination.

The test should be acceptable to the population.

Treatment

There should be an accepted treatment for patients with recognized disease.

Screening Program

There should be an established policy on whom to treat as patients.

Facilities for diagnosis and treatment should be available. The cost of case finding, including diagnosis and treatment, should be economically balanced in relation to possible expenditure on medical care as a whole.

Case finding should be a continuing process and not a "once and for all" project.

Source: Wilson JM, Junger GG. Principles and practice of screening for disease. World Health Organization Public Health Papers, No. 34; 1968.

The screening test should be sufficiently accurate to detect the disease at an early stage.

There must be a treatment for the disease. It is unethical to initiate a screening program if the treatment required to act on the results is not available.

Early detection should lead to improved survival.

Facilities for diagnosis and treatment must be available.

The screening test should be acceptable to the target population.

The screening test should be cost-effective.

The screening test should be sufficiently sensitive and specific.

The ethical imperative for all medical interventions is to ensure as far as possible that the potential benefits will outweigh the potential harms.

Limitations of Screening

Several pitfalls in screening must be taken into account. In particular, two types of errors can and do occur: the test result may incorrectly show a positive result when in fact the individual does not have the disease (false positive), and conversely, the test may be negative when in fact the individual does have the disease (false negative). Other limitations of screening programs are stress and anxiety caused by the false positive screening test result; unnecessary investigation and treatment of false-positive results; the cost of further diagnostic testing/workup; and a false sense of security caused by false negatives, which may end up delaying diagnosis and treatment. Weighing the potential benefits of the screening program against the potential harms is imperative.

Screening also may lead to overdiagnosis and overtreatment, which would not have posed a problem to the individual had the screening test not identified the "problem." *Overdiagnosis* refers to "disease" that will almost never cause symptoms or death during a patient's lifetime. These conditions are referred to as "harmless abnormalities." That is, some cancers are slow growing and best left alone, but if a screening test is positive, there is an ethical mandate to order tests to diagnose the problem definitively, which often leads to unnecessary, costly treatment.

The effectiveness of early treatment is among one of the more important factors to consider when deciding whether or not to screen. If effective treatment is not available, ethically one should not screen for the disease in the first place. For a screening program to be beneficial (to improve health outcomes or increase life expectancy), it must include a treatment that is not only effective but also *more effective* if applied earlier rather than later. If the treatment works just as well later in the course of the disease, screening for early detection is not necessary.

Lead time and length time bias are two issues that also need to be taken into account when assessing the impact of a screening program. *Lead time bias* refers to the length of time between the detection of a disease and its clinical presentation and diagnosis. It is the period between early diagnosis with screening and when diagnosis would have been made without screening. That is, the disease is detected earlier in its natural history with screening. Survival appears to be increased because the disease is detected earlier in the natural history. The *survival time since diagnosis* is longer with screening; but *life span* is not prolonged. Screening appears to increase survival time (lead time), but those with the disease, whether they were screened or not, die at the same time.

Length time bias is often discussed in the context of the benefits of cancer screening. It occurs when disease detected by screening is less aggressive than disease detected without screening, which can lead to the perception that screening leads to better outcomes when in reality it has no effect. For example, breast cancers detected in a screening program may be less aggressive than those diagnosed when symptoms appear. Less-aggressive cancers grow slower; therefore the length of time that a cancer is detectable by screening is greater for the slow-growing tumors. People whose cancer is detected by screening may appear to live longer because their cancers grow at a slower pace. That is, slower-growing tumors have better prognoses than tumors with faster-growing tumors. Screening is more likely to detect slower-growing tumors, which may be less deadly than faster-growing tumors. Thus screening may tend to detect cancers that would not have killed the patient or even been detected prior to death from other causes. Figure 2.1 illustrates lead time and length time bias.

Cancer Screening

It is a commonly held belief among health professionals that early diagnosis of cancer is beneficial and that therefore screening should be implemented. The thinking is that when cancer is detected at an early stage, there should be a reduction in mortality; the prognosis for survival should be better than if there were no screening. The cancer would be "caught early," thus increasing the likelihood that people would not die from the disease. In addition to the factors discussed previously, an individual's quality of life must be taken into account, especially when thinking about screening for specific cancers. The quality-adjusted life year (QALY) is a measure of the state of health of a person or group in which the benefits, in terms of length of life, are adjusted to reflect the quality of life. The QALY is a widely used measure of health improvement that is used to guide health care resource allocation decisions, and it assumes that health or health improvement can be measured or valued based on amounts of time spent in various health states.

Over the years considerable debate and discussion have focused on the questions of which cancers to screen, on which population, at what age, and how frequently. Consider a woman in her early forties with an average risk

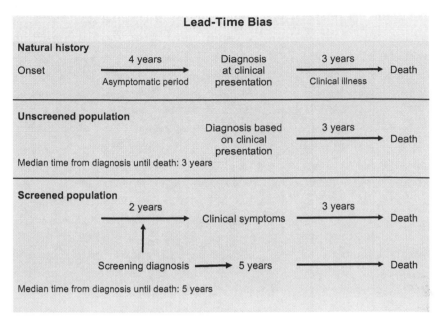

Figure 2.1. Diagram of Lead Time and Length Time Bias

of breast cancer. Should she have a mammogram annually? Every two years? Not until age fifty? Naturally she would want to have a cancer detected at an early stage. However, there has been much controversy regarding the age at which routine mammography screening should begin. Although the data do not provide a clear indication that screening women at younger ages (such as less than fifty years of age) is beneficial, clearly many factors (such as genetic, demographic, personal, biology of the disease, and patient preference) need to be taken into account when making the decision.

More recently there has been controversy about whether prostate-specific antigen (PSA) screening should be used at all in men. As with breast cancer, many factors must be taken into account in deciding who would benefit from PSA screening. The sensitivity and specificity of the test need to be considered. As a rule, anyone who tests positive on a screening test must be worked-up further, and this usually involves invasive testing and the concomitant costs. In addition, the potential harm (in this case risk of impotence or incontinence should prostate surgery be performed) should be balanced against the potential benefits. Would doing nothing be a better course of action? The importance of data must be stressed. What do the screening studies show about the potential benefits and potential risks of a screening test?

However, there are several types of cancer for which the potential benefits of screening outweigh the potential risks or harm of not detecting the cancer at an early stage. The cases presented in this book focus primarily on two cancers, cervical and oral. Both are highly prevalent in low- and middle-income countries (LMICs), and there are screening tests for them that are easy to administer and do not cost very much. But most important, detecting these cancers at an early stage makes a difference in survival. Screening for other cancers, such as breast, prostate, and colorectal, is the norm in the developed world, but huge challenges remain in LMICs despite the fact that the incidence and mortality of these cancers are high. As discussed in chapter 1, it is not feasible to undertake population-based screening in LIMCs for most cancers. The exceptions are cervical and oral cavity cancer. Following is a brief overview of the feasibility, benefits, and challenges of screening for these cancers in LMICs.

Cervical Cancer Screening

Cervical cancer, a relatively slow-growing cancer, is the fourth leading cause of death among women worldwide, but the leading cause of cancer mortality among women living in LMICs. (1) Cervical cancer remains one of the leading causes of death in women, especially women in sub-Saharan Africa, South America, and Southeast Asia, including India. There is striking global health inequity, resulting in higher morbidity and mortality among women living in LMICs than women living in the developed world. These women, mothers, wives, and grandmothers, are in their most productive years of life and contribute economically to family welfare. Their deaths leave a large gap in the fabric of the family. The evidence from numerous studies shows that most of the cases of cervical cancer deaths could have been prevented had the women been screened and the disease detected at an early stage. Cervical cancer is both preventable and curable if diagnosed in its early stage.

Of the known risk factors for cervical cancer, human papillomavirus (HPV) infection has been shown to be the primary risk factor, as HPV is found in the overwhelming majority of cases of cervical cancer. That being said, while HPV infection is necessary for the development of cervical neoplasia, the vast majority of women infected with HPV do not develop cervical cancer. In most women, HPV infections are usually transient. The risk of cervical cancer, however, increases with the number of lifetime sex partners, early sexual activity, frequency of reinfection, and intratypic genetic variation within HPV type. (2)

There are approximately one hundred types of HPV, with variations in their genetic and oncogenic potential, most of which are considered low risk and do not lead to cervical cancer. However, there are high-risk HPV types (e.g., HPV 16 and 18) that are responsible for approximately 70 percent of cervical cancers. Testing for high-risk HPV types is now being used to screen for cervical cancer, even in LIMCs. HPV testing relies on molecular-biology techniques, which allow for accurate detection and typing. HPV DNA testing is a screening modality designed to detect precancerous lesions and can easily be used in a "screen and treat" setting. It has been demonstrated to be a cost-effective way to reduce cervical cancer incidence. (3)

Qiagen's careHPV test, a rapid, highly sensitive DNA test appropriate for use in LIMCs, detects the DNA of fourteen types of the HPV that cause cervical cancer. This test can also be effectively used even in very basic clinics, and its sensitivity is comparable to that of Pap testing (i.e., careHPV detects more infection with HPV). The Digene hybrid capture 2 high risk HPV DNA Test (HC2) is another highly sensitive and specific test for HPV DNA detection (sensitivity 93.3% and specificity: 97%). The concordance rate between careHPV and HC2 has been shown to be excellent: 93.81%. (4) Polymerase chain reaction (PCR) DNA testing is also a standard, noninvasive method for determining the presence of a cervical HPV infection. (For more in-depth discussion of various HPV DNA tests, see Abreu [5].)

Newer technologies allow for self-collection of HPV test samples; a woman can collect vaginal samples in the comfort of her home. There is no need for a trained health care provider or pelvic exam. The woman packages the sample in a specially designed collection packet, which is deposited at a dedicated collection site for analysis. Self-testing has been shown to have similar sensitivity (83.3%) to that of clinic collection. HPV self-screening could help overcome cultural barriers to gynecological visits and enable physicians and nurses to focus on providing medical services to those in need. Evidence shows that a single negative HPV DNA test provides five to ten years of confidence against a high-grade precancerous cervical lesion. (6) The WHO has endorsed visual inspection with acetic acid (VIA) and HPV testing as acceptable cervical cancer screening modalities in LMICs. (7)

Chapter 3 provides a comprehensive overview of HPV infection and its role in cervical cancer. It discusses the benefits and limitations of HPV DNA testing in conjunction with or in lieu of VIA testing. The HPV DNA test is sufficiently sensitive and specific and is easy to administer. The cost, however, could be a barrier in some settings. This chapter also presents the pros and cons of HPV vaccination. HPV vaccine has the potential to be a game-changer in the effort to prevent cervical cancer, in that the vaccine is an important measure to block HPV transmission and to prevent cervical cancer. Three vaccines are currently available in the United States: Gardasil (marketed by Merck), Gardasil 9 (an HPV 9-valent vaccine, recombinant, marketed by Merck), and Cervarix (marketed by Glaxo Smith Kline). All three vaccines prevent infections with HPV types 16 and 18. The FDA has approved Gardasil and Gardasil 9 for use in females nine through twenty-six years old for the prevention of HPV-caused cervical, vulvar, vaginal, and anal cancers; precancerous cervical, vulvar, vaginal, and anal lesions; and genital warts. Gardasil and Gardasil 9 are also approved for use in males for the prevention of HPV-caused anal cancer, precancerous anal lesions, and genital warts. Gardasil is approved for use in males nine through twenty-six years old, and Gardasil 9 is approved for use in males nine through fifteen years old. Cervarix is approved for use in females nine through twenty-five years old for the prevention of HPV-caused cervical cancer.

Two vaccines are available globally: a quadrivalent vaccine (Gardasil) and a bivalent vaccine (Cervarix). Both are manufactured by recombinant DNA technology. Vaccination is recommended prior to the onset of sexual activity. None of the case studies included in this book discusses an ongoing vaccination program, primarily because of governmental challenges. However, all of the authors tout the benefits of HPV vaccination and call for widespread immunization.

Many of the case studies presented in this book discuss innovative ways to screen for cervical cancer in LMICs, especially in rural, poor areas of the world. As the reader will discern, there are many different ways to screen for cervical cancer. All of the programs rely on low-tech means to screen (such as VIA) because the Pap test and other cervical cytology screening methods are not feasible in rural settings. These tests require skilled physicians and cytologists and a cytology lab. VIA, on the other hand, can be performed by a trained health care worker (not necessarily a physician). This individual is taught how to visualize with the naked eye precancerous cervical lesions. Results are immediate, the test is cost effective, and a woman can be referred for treatment immediately (screen and treat). The VIA test has been shown repeatedly to be competitively sensitive and specific compared to the gold standard, the Pap test. This is fortunate because, as mentioned previously, the Pap test and other cervical cytology screening methods are usually not feasible in rural settings.

Chapter 4 focuses on a cervical cancer screening program that serves rural, poor women in Tamil Nadu, India. The Rural Unit of Health and Social Affairs (RUHSA) provides primary and secondary level health care to over 138,000 people. In 2007 RUHSA introduced its "Educate, Screen, and Treat" program for cervical cancer with the aim of providing early detection, treatment, and education. One of the essential activities of the program is to screen women between the ages of thirty and fifty using VIA. Public health nurses and physicians screen women in eighteen outreach clinics. All women who test positive are referred to the secondary level community health center at RUHSA, where a second VIA test is done for confirmation. Cryotherapy can be done at RUHSA, but women who require more advanced care are referred to the tertiary hospital in Vellore. The health education and awareness program is an important component of the screening program. Lack of awareness about cervical cancer is something that the RUHSA staff work on every day.

More than 6,600 women were screened. The biggest challenge has been how to encourage women who test positive to seek treatment. Most do not follow up with necessary care. Part of the problem is the inability to pay for follow-up care. The authors of chapter 4 call on the Indian government to step up its efforts in helping to defray the costs of screening and treatment.

Chapter 5 discusses a screen and treat program in rural Malawi, a country with one of the world's highest rates of cervical cancer. It shares the successes (huge interest among the target population and a high detection rate of cervical cancer) and limitations (logistical/transportation issues, poor awareness of the disease, and costs) of the Nkhoma Hospital cervical cancer screening program. The program relied on VIA; for those who tested positive, thermo-coagulation (an ablative method for treatment of cervical intraepithelial neoplasia) was introduced as a replacement for cryotherapy. The equipment for thermos-coagulation is easily portable and durable. Importantly, the efficacy of treatment of lesions with thermos-coagulation was comparable to that of cryotherapy.

Screening for cervical cancer is a huge challenge in resource-poor Haiti. In chapter 6 researchers from Innovating Health International (IHI) share their problems and challenges in setting up a screening program in Haiti. Working with Haiti sans Cervical Cancer, a loose collection of nongovernmental organizations, they designed a "prevent and treat" cervical cancer network. They relied on VIA and cryotherapy in eight of the largest hospitals, located in the geographic departments of Haiti. Challenges include the paucity of OB-GYN physicians, a substandard transportation network, financial barriers, lack of awareness, and little ability to provide follow-up treatment (e.g., there is no option for radiation therapy in Haiti). In cooperation with the Haitian Support Group Against Cancer and other local partners, IHI implemented a women's cancer awareness and engagement campaign. However, if follow-up treatment is not available or too costly, is it ethical to screen?

Chapter 7 focuses on PCR testing for high-risk HPV in Honduras. The program described in this chapter shows the importance of working with local groups and the government to achieve success. A team approach, one that fostered collaborative team science, formed the basis of an ambitious screening program in rural and urban parts of the country. The mass screening programs are beautifully described and can serve as a guide for others seeking to implement cancer screening programs in LMICs. The team relied on VIA as well as high-risk HPV screening using molecular methods to help alleviate the need for Pap smear testing. The authors stress that the key to their program's success was the grassroots relationships among investigators, local clinicians, and village residents. They have created the groundwork for a sustained high-risk HPV screening program and hopefully a pathway that will reduce cervical cancer mortality in Honduran women.

Oral Cancer Screening

While cancers of the breast, cervix, colon, and prostate are the focus of most cancer prevention screening programs, the relatively high incidence of oral cavity cancer, particularly in LMICs, highlights the need for screening and treatment as well as for prevention initiatives. The annual estimated global incidence is approximately 275,000 for oral and 130,300 for oropharyngeal cancers (excluding nasopharynx), with two-thirds of these cases occurring in developing countries. (8) There is a wide geographical variation (approximately twenty-fold) in the incidence of this cancer. Countries with the highest rates of oral cavity cancer are found in South and Southeast Asia (e.g., Sri Lanka, India, Pakistan, and Taiwan), parts of Western (e.g., France) and Eastern Europe (e.g., Hungary, Slovakia, and Slovenia), parts of Latin America and the Caribbean (e.g., Brazil, Uruguay, and Puerto Rico), and the Pacific region (e.g., Papua New Guinea and Melanesia). (8)

Oropharyngeal cancers (cancers of the middle part of the throat, including the soft palate, the base of the tongue, and the tonsils) generally have a poor prognosis, primarily because most cases are diagnosed in the advanced stages despite the fact that it is a preventable form of cancer and easily treatable when diagnosed in the early stages. Viruses, in particular the HPV and herpes simplex virus (HSV), have been linked to oropharyngeal cancers. About 70 percent of oropharyngeal cancers are caused by HPV, the overwhelming majority of which is HPV16. (9)

Tobacco use, alcohol consumption, and areca nut chewing are considered to be the primary risk factors for this type of cancer. The early signs of oropharyngeal cancers can easily be overlooked, as they generally are not painful. That being said, early warning symptoms include persistent white and/or red patches in the oral cavity, nonhealing ulcers, noticeable surface changes, tooth mobility with no apparent cause, atypical bleeding in the oral or nasal cavity, and prolonged hoarseness. Symptoms commonly seen in late stages include pain or difficulty in swallowing, speaking, or chewing; any wart-like masses; hoarseness that lasts for a long time; any numbness in the oral/facial region; and enlargement of the lymph nodes. Generally, it is in the later stages that persistent pain will be reported, alongside some or all of these symptoms. (10) The overall five-year survival rate for oropharyngeal cancers is approximately 50 percent, with best outcomes for cancer of the lip (90% survival rate). (11)

Early diagnosis and treatment could influence survival, but many other factors must be taken into account, such as lifestyle, treatment modality, and stage of the tumor. Chapter 8, dealing with oral cancer screening, describes the challenges in organizing and administering a screening program in LMICs. This chapter presents a comprehensive discussion of the benefits and challenges of screening for oral cancer. Despite the high prevalence and high mortality of oral cancers, especially in LMICs, few countries that have implemented national oral cancer screening programs. The authors provide a balanced review, outlining the evidence base for the screening of oral cancer and oral potentially malignant disorders (OPMDs) in LMICs, using the criteria from the UK National Screening Committee as a "gold" standard to assess whether the evidence supports oral cancer screening.

Breast Cancer Screening

Breast cancer is a leading cause of death and disability among women in both high- and low-income countries. Though incidence and overall mortality rates in LMICs are lower than in most high-income countries, case fatality rates from breast cancer are very high in LMICs, primarily because of lack of screening and a scarcity of adequate facilities for detection and treatment. (12) More than half of incident cases occur in the developing world. (13) Mammography is the primary means of screening for breast cancer in the developed world; however, there are downsides to this technology. A seventeen-year study on Danish women concluded that screening mammography does not reduce the incidence of advanced tumors, but does increase the diagnosis of lesions that would not become cancers needing treatment. (14) One would have expected that screening would have reduced the incidence of advanced tumors and increased survival, but this was not the case. Breast cancer mortality is not lowered. Other studies have shown similar findings. (15) Therefore, the value of mammography is being questioned by many researchers.

While mammography, other expensive technologies, and therapies are not likely to be available in LMICs, clinical breast exams performed by health care providers can help identify women with breast abnormalities that would require diagnostic workup. Education about breast cancer, coupled with early detection and timely, adequate surgery, could result in substantial improvements in survival in much of the developing world. However, in many places radiation therapy and chemotherapy are not available, or if available, are too costly for most of those in need. That being said, benefits can be realized from basic breast cancer education and awareness campaigns. Breast exams should be integrated into the primary health care infrastructure, with treatment modalities (usually a mastectomy) expanded to meet the need.

Given the high incidence and case fatality of breast cancer in LMICs, doing nothing should not be an option. There is an important role for improving breast cancer awareness among the general population in LMICs as well as among primary care practitioners. This could be the first step in setting up an early detection program. Early detection to improve breast cancer outcome and survival remains the cornerstone of breast cancer control and should be made available to women in LMICs.

Prostate Cancer Screening

If detected by screening in its very early stages prostate cancer, a slow-growing malignancy, can often be effectively treated. While prevalent in the developed world, it is less so in LMICs, perhaps because of the lack of screening for this cancer and/or the paucity of valid data showing the incidence and prevalence. Compounding the issue, there is a great deal of controversy surrounding the role of prostate cancer screening in the reduction of mortality. Typical screening modalities include the PSA test and digital rectal exam (DRE); however, the reliability of the PSA test has been called into question because the test doesn't always provide an accurate result. An elevated PSA level doesn't necessarily mean the individual has cancer. And many men diagnosed with prostate cancer have a normal PSA level. Until there is a sensitive and specific test for prostate cancer, it is doubtful that screening programs will be implemented in LMICs.

Colon and Rectal Screening

Colorectal cancer is the third most common cancer in men, and the fourth most common in women. (8) There is considerable variation in the incidence of colorectal cancer among regions of the world. Although it is more prevalent in the developed world, mortality in the LMICs is much higher primarily because of a lack of screening for the cancer. Mortality is related to survival of colorectal cancer, which depends on the proportion of early detection and curative treatment. While colonoscopies are the mainstay of colon cancer screening in the developed world, most LMICs would not be able to implement such a screening program. The costs are prohibitive, and the acceptance of this invasive test among the population could be a huge challenge/barrier. However, the fecal occult blood test (FOBT) is a somewhat sensitive and specific test for colorectal cancer and can be administered easily and inexpensively. For those who test positive, a flexible sigmoidoscopy or colonoscopy, the gold standard procedure for the early detection of colorectal cancer and premalignant adenomatous polyps, would be warranted, but in many LMICs, particularly in rural areas, these tests are all but impossible to do.

Lambert, Sauvaget, and Sankaranarayanan (16) have argued that the expense of mounting a mass screening effort in most LMICs is not currently justified given the significant costs of colonoscopy and follow-up services. A prudent course of action would be for LMICs to implement an educational awareness campaign focusing on the risk factors of colorectal cancer and prevention.

Harnessing Technology

Reliance on mobile technology is an exciting avenue to pursue. Billions of people live in remote rural communities around the world and receive little or no medical care. Mobile technology is the fastest growing technology in human history, reaching and connecting more people in developing countries than ever before. I have heard it said that there are more mobile phones in India than toilets! Over 97 percent of the global population now lives within reach of a mobile phone signal.

Chapter 9 presents a compelling overview of the advantages of mHealth, including how technology can be harnessed to provide education and information quickly and easily and how it can be used in data collection to evaluate programs, as is the case in the cervical cancer screening program described in chapter 4. Chapter 9 reports that one of the most common uses of mHealth is to facilitate communication among patients, health workers, and facility-based care providers, particularly when access to treatment is limited, costly, or difficult, as is the case in many LMICs.

The Need for Palliative Care

It is unrealistic to expect that screening will prevent all cancers from advancing to late-stage disease and death. The need for a plan to care for the dying is an integral component of disease management. Chapter 10 explores palliative care, arguing that it affords everyone a dignified, compassionate way to die and should be as important as screening for the disease in the first place. Every palliative care program needs to be flexible, adapt to changing needs of the community, and respect the local norms and mores related to death and dying. Helping people die a "good death" by means of palliative care, even in LMICs, is indeed not only feasible but also necessary.

Conclusion

The goal of cancer screening is to detect cancer or precancerous lesions in asymptomatic individuals at a point when cancer is more likely to be prevented or cured than if the patient waited for symptoms to develop. Implicit is that effective treatment for early-stage disease must be available, affordable, and acceptable. For many reasons, delayed presentation of cancer is the norm in many LMICs: lack of awareness among the population; lack of trained personnel; lack of facilities, including pathology labs; logistical issues, including poor transportation, that make appropriate care inaccessible or impossible; lack of treatment for disease management for those who are diagnosed with the cancer; and lack of funds to pay for screening and treatment. Organized approaches to screening risk increasing the burden on already shaky health care systems. Above all else, there needs to be a mechanism in place to refer individuals who test positive at screening for follow-up treatment. If this is not feasible, then the value of screening needs to be assessed. If there are few resources in place for follow-up care (such as money, trained providers, and appropriate diagnostic equipment), then screening probably should not be undertaken. Similarly, ethical considerations must be taken into account before a screening program is offered. The benefits of screening must outweigh its potential harm.

The joint report of the World Economic Forum/Harvard School of Public Health and the World Health Organization highlights a set of affordable, feasible, and cost-effective intervention strategies to reduce the economic impact of non-communicable diseases in LMICs. (17) The report concludes that breast and cervical cancer screening are recommended as first cancer screening priorities in those countries. Ultimately, the success of a cancer screening program depends on the willingness of the public to take part in the screening process. This in turn depends to a great extent on how the benefits and risks of the procedure are communicated. Developing a screening policy for cancer is complex and involves many decisions at the local and state levels. The following chapters describe the challenges of implementing a cancer screening program in several LMICs.

References

1. Ferlay J, Soerjomataram I, Dikshit R, et al. Cancer incidence and mortality worldwide: sources, methods and major patterns in GLOBOCAN 2012. Int J Cancer 2015;136: E359–86.

2. Gomez, DT, Santos, JL. Human papillomavirus infection and cervical cancer: pathogenesis and epidemiology. In: Vilas Menez A, editor. Communicating current research and educational topics and trends in applied microbiology. Vol 2. Babajoz, Spain: FORMATEX; 2004. p. 680–8.

3. Schiffman M, Castle PE. The promise of global cervical cancer prevention. N Engl J Med 2005;353(20):2101–4.

4. Ying H, Jing F, Fanghui Z, et al. High-risk HPV nucleic acid detection kit—the careHPV test—a new detection method for screening. Sci Rep 2014;4:4704. doi: 10.1038/srep04704.

5. Abreu AL et al. A review of methods for detect human Papillomavirus infection. Virol J 2012;9:26. doi.org/10.1186/1743-422X-9-262.

6. Sherman ME, Lorinca AT, Scott DR, et al. Baseline cytology, human papillomavirus testing, and risk for cervical neoplasia: a 10-year cohort analysis. J Natl Cancer Inst 2003;95:46–52.

7. Guidelines for screening and treatment of precancerous lesions for cervical cancer prevention 2013 [cited 2016 Dec 20]. Available from: http://apps.who.int/rhl /guidelines/screening_and_treatment_of_precancerous_lesions/en/.

8. Ferlay J, Pisani P, Parkin DM. GLOBOCAN 2002: cancer incidence, mortality, and prevalence worldwide. IARC Cancer Base (2002 estimates). Lyon: IARC Press; 2004.

9. Shillitoe, EJ. The role of viruses in squamous cell carcinoma of the oropharyngeal mucosa. Oral Oncol 2009;45:351–5.

10. Oral cancer facts [cited 2015 Jul 8]. Available from: http://www.oralcancer foundation.org/facts/.

11. Warnakulasuriya, S. Global epidemiology of oral and oropharyngeal cancer. Oral Oncol 2009;45:309–316.

12. Shulman LM, Willett W, Sievers A, et al. Breast cancer in developing countries: opportunities for improved survival. J Oncol 2010;2010:595167.

13. Beaulieu N, Bloom D, Bloom R, Stein R. Breakaway: the global burden of cancer—challenges and opportunities. London: The Economist Intelligence Unit; 2009.

14. Jørgensen KJ, Gøtzsche PC, Kalager M, et al. Breast cancer screening in Denmark: a cohort study of tumor size and overdiagnosis. Ann Int Med 2017.doi: 10.7326/M16–0270.

15. Miller AB, Wall C, Baines CJ, et al. Twenty five year follow-up for breast cancer incidence and mortality of the Canadian National Breast Screening Study: randomised screening trial. BMJ 2014;348:g366. doi: http://dx.doi.org/10.1136/bmj .g366.

16. Lambert R, Sauvaget C, Sankaranarayanan R. Mass screening for colorectal cancer is not justified in most developing countries. Int J Cancer 2009;125:253–6.

17. World Economic Forum. From burden to best buys: Reducing the economic impact of non-communicable disease in low and middle-income countries. Geneva, Switzerland: WEF; 2011 [cited 2015 Jul 8]. Available from: http://www.who.int/nmh /publications/best_buys_summary.pdf.

Chapter 3

Shobha S. Krishnan

Challenges in Screening for Cervical Cancer

Sharing Experiences from India

*The difference between what we do, and what we
are capable of doing, would suffice to solve most of
the world's problems.* — *Mohandas Gandhi*

L ife has an uncanny knack of redirecting one's destiny. Like most people, I
had plans and dreams laid out for myself, but what came to me instead—an
opportunity to fight cervical cancer—turned out to be a better path
than I ever could have planned for myself. This journey began in the
summer of 2008 with the publication of my book, *The HPV Vaccine Controversy: Sex, Cancer, God, and Politics.* During a vacation I took in Kutch,
a remote area in the northwest part of Gujarat, India, a woman who was
struggling with disease said, "I just heard you say that India has the highest
number of cervical cancer deaths in the world and that one young woman
is dying from this disease every 7 to 8 minutes in this country. What are
you going to do about it?" Her plea, her challenge, galvanized me to "do
something about it."

I established a nongovernmental organization (NGO) called Global Initiative Against HPV and Cervical Cancer (GIAHC), with the mission to try
to save lives from cervical cancer, one woman at a time, one day at a time.
Our goals are to build relationships to develop, strengthen, and support
HPV and cervical cancer prevention, screening, and treatment programs;
develop culturally sensitive and linguistically appropriate health education
materials to promote healthy living; co-host screening training workshops
on a periodic basis to train local community health workers (physicians,
nurses, and other qualified health personnel); and identify barriers to help

communities implement creative, medically sound, economically sustainable, and practical solutions for effective management of screening and early treatment. We focused on India because of the great unmet need there to address screening for this disease.

The objective of this chapter is to describe how a grassroots organization with a specific purpose can make a difference in people's lives. The discussion highlights the barriers we faced and the impact we have had on women's lives.

HPV Background

Nearly all cases of cervical cancer can be attributed to human papillomavirus (HPV) infection. As chapter 2 discussed, HPV plays a major role in the development of cervical cancer. There are more than one hundred types of HPV, of which at least thirteen are cancer causing (also known as high-risk type). These types of HPV can cause oral, penile, and anal cancers in men and cervical, vaginal, vulvar, oral, and anal cancers in women. The low-risk types cause genital warts, which are highly contagious. Identifying specific HPV types that are strongly associated with cervical cancer was an important step in the fight against cervical cancer. In 2008 the Nobel Prize for Medicine was awarded to three virologists, one of whom, Dr. Harald Zur Hausen from Germany, won for the detection and isolation of HPV types 16 and 18. These are the major precursors of almost all cervical cancers, and they are detected in approximately 70 percent of cervical cancers. (1)

The HPV virus spreads both nonsexually (through genital-to-genital or hand-to-genital contact) and sexually (through vaginal or anal intercourse), with sexual activity comprising the most common form of transmission. (2) The peak time for acquiring infection for both women and men is shortly after becoming sexually active. Most sexually active women and men will be infected at some point in their lives, and some may be repeatedly infected. (3) Risk factors for HPV infection include early first sexual intercourse, multiple sexual partners, tobacco use, and immune suppression. HIV-infected individuals are at higher risk of HPV infection and are infected by a broader range of HPV types. It takes on average fifteen to twenty years for cervical cancer to develop in women with normal immune systems, but for women with weakened immune systems, the time period can be much shorter. (3)

Although most HPV infections clear up on their own, and most precancerous lesions resolve spontaneously, there is a risk that HPV infection may become chronic and that precancerous lesions could progress to invasive cervical cancer. Having an HPV infection, however, does not mean that a person will automatically develop disease or even cancer. HPV is a silent infection, and most people who become infected do not know that they have been infected. HPV infection also runs a very unpredictable course. It can be contracted through a partner without any symptoms, remain dormant, and then unknowingly be transmitted to the next partner.

One of the "best" ways to prevent the development of advanced cervical cancer is to screen for the disease. Cervical cancer is easily detected by various screening modalities; if it is identified at an early stage, the prognosis is excellent. Screening is most effective for women between the ages of thirty and forty-nine, when it has the potential for the greatest impact. Cervical cancer is not common among women younger than thirty years of age, and therefore screening is not recommended for them. The World Health Organization (WHO) recommends targeting screening to women who are between thirty and forty-nine years old because of their higher risk for developing cervical cancer. (4)

Screening Methods Most Suited for Rural India

In rural areas of developing countries, it is next to impossible to conduct a cervical cancer screening using the Pap smear, the gold standard test in the developed world. Many developing countries such as India lack high-quality cytology labs and trained technicians to read the slides. The cost of the test is usually more than a woman can afford. In addition, in India the overwhelming majority of the population live in villages, some at great distances from health centers or hospitals. Hence trying to develop and maintain a screening program using the Pap smear is just not feasible in these areas. We therefore had to be creative and innovative in our approach to designing a cervical cancer screening program in rural India. We had to find a sensitive, specific, cost-effective test that could be administered in rural areas. Fortunately such a test exists and has been used successfully in many developing countries.

Visual inspection with acetic acid (VIA) has been shown repeatedly to be an excellent alternative to cytology-based screening programs in developing countries. (5–7) Essentially, VIA relies on vinegar, a product that is readily available even in rural areas. In this procedure, the cervix is painted with vinegar (3–5% acetic acid). Normal cervical tissue remains unaffected by the acetic acid, but the excess DNA protein found in abnormal tissue coagulates in the presence of vinegar and turns white. Women with the telltale white areas need to undergo additional testing to rule out or diagnosis cervical cancer. In many instances the woman can be treated at the time of screening by cryotherapy (freezing the cells with a probe using liquid nitrogen or carbon dioxide). This method of using VIA followed by cryotherapy was pioneered in the 1990s by physicians working in Africa and India and was later endorsed by the WHO.

The WHO endorsement specifically came from a demonstration project that was conducted in six African countries (Madagascar, Malawi, Nigeria, Uganda, United Republic of Tanzania, and Zambia) between 2005 and 2009. (8) It showed that VIA is a viable alternative to cytology-based screening in low-resource settings; the sensitivity of the VIA test is comparable to that of the Pap smear, although with a slightly lower specificity. The WHO concluded that VIA was simple, safe, feasible, and acceptable to women and providers in low-resource settings. (9) For those who test positive, cryotherapy is the treatment of choice, assuming that providers of care know how to treat using this therapy.

Visual inspection with acetic acid is a cheap and quick procedure that does not require lab processing or electricity, making it ideally suited for low- and middle-income countries, especially rural areas. In addition, VIA is well-suited for task shifting, as it can be effectively taught to nurses and community health workers. It does not have to be performed by a physician. Workshops lasting between two days and two weeks can effectively train allied health personnel to perform VIA. Our NGO has participated in training sessions, in which trainees pore over slides and flash cards showing cervixes with diagnosable problems, then practice cryotherapy on sliced sausages inserted inside plastic tubes. "It is a simple test that nurses and trained community health care providers can administer," one nurse said. "The patient lies down to be examined, the cervix is washed with vinegar[;] if it turns white, it means it is a positive test and I freeze it. There are minimal side effects. If I am in doubt, I refer her to the doctor."

In our screening program we, like other NGOs, have found that there is a learning curve after the VIA training session. New trainees have approximately twice the number of positive VIAs (around 30%) as veterans (around 15%). (10,11) In their desire not to miss any potentially positive cases, new trainees have a tendency to identify benign cellular changes such as squamous metaplasia as positive, which probably accounts for the higher numbers of positive cases among the new trainees. However, we have found that within six to twelve months, with a trained eye, the new trainees become more confident and accurate in their interpretation of positive and negative cases.

The "screen and treat" protocol using VIA allows women to get their test results immediately, thus obviating the need to have an individual return to the clinic days or weeks later or to have the clinic staff travel into the villages to find her. Those who test positive can have cryotherapy on the spot. These "one-stop" or "single-visit" programs are based on the fundamental principle that fewer women will be lost to follow-up care if they can receive treatment during the same visit in which they are screened.

While low-tech screening options such as the VIA have many advantages, there are some limitations, which can lead to overtreatment of women who screen positive. For example, there is subjectivity in differentiating benign from malignant test results; the results may vary depending on how well the screener was trained. There is an issue of low specificity and reduced reliability in women fifty years of age or older because the squamo-columnar junction recedes into the endocervical canal in menopausal women, making it more difficult to detect cancer. (12)

The strong association between cervical cancer and HPV makes testing for the genetic material of HPV a valuable screening tool. A new test (the HPV DNA test), designed to detect the genetic material of the virus, has been developed. It is accurate, objective, and easy to administer. The test has a comparatively higher sensitivity (94.6–96.1%) and specificity (90.7–94.1%) than cytology or VIA. (13) In addition, women do not need to undergo frequent screening. (14) The test can be performed on cervical or vaginal samples. The advantage of vaginal samples is that a woman can take her own vaginal swab in the privacy of her home. Many studies have shown that self-testing is well accepted by women and can improve compliance. (15) In addition, self-collected samples have been shown to produce comparable performance to clinician-collected HPV samples. (16–19) This strategy may reduce the infrastructure requirements inherent in other screening options.

Probably the biggest limitation of the HPV DNA test, however, is that it requires a sophisticated laboratory and trained technicians, and it takes four to seven hours to process the specimen. In comparison to the VIA, with its immediate results, this could be an issue in some areas. It also is a comparatively expensive test. To make the HPV DNA test simpler, more affordable, faster, and more feasible for low-resource settings, a rapid molecular test for

HPV (careHPV) has been developed. (20) The rapid HPV DNA test is portable, is simpler to perform, and allows for field interpretation of the results within two and one-half hours, without any requirement for electricity or running water. It has proven to be a feasible test for use in rural areas. (21)

Our organization is currently working with partners in rural India who are performing the VIA test followed by cryotherapy. Yet there is considerable enthusiasm to introduce the rapid molecular HPV DNA test. The price of the test, the cost of the machine needed to process the samples, and the design of its packaging, with ninety-six test wells to a tray, make it suitable for use in camp settings, where many women can be screened at one arranged time. However, if this were to be used as a part of one-stop screen and treat program, the logistical challenges of having ninety-six women waiting at the screening site for more than two hours while the tests were being processed, then treating the positive cases on the same day, would require considerable human resources and time. Hence we are currently at the crossroads of introducing this new technology and weighing the feasibility and sustainability of doing so.

Denny et al. (22) conducted a randomized screening trial using the hybrid capture 2 HPV DNA test and VIA to evaluate the safety, acceptability, and efficacy of these two screen and treat approaches through thirty-six months of follow-up. The study sample consisted of 6,555 South African women thirty-five to sixty-five years old who were tested for the presence of high-risk HPV DNA in cervical samples. The women underwent visual inspection of the cervix using acetic acid staining and HIV serotesting. They were randomly assigned to three study arms: (1) HPV-and-treat, in which all women with a positive HPV DNA test result underwent cryotherapy; (2) visual inspection-and-treat, in which all women with a positive visual inspection test result underwent cryotherapy; and (3) control, in which further evaluation or treatment was delayed for six months. All the women underwent colposcopy with biopsy at six months. The findings show that after thirty-six months, there was a sustained, statistically significant decrease in the cumulative detection of cervical intraepithelial neoplasia grade 2+ (CIN2+) in the HPV-and-treat arm compared with the control arm (1.5% vs 5.6%, 95% confidence interval 2.8% to 5.3%). The HPV screen and treat arm was associated with a 3.7-fold reduction in the cumulative detection of CIN2+ over a thirty-six-month period of follow-up. The VIA treatment arm showed a 1.5-fold reduction. The researchers concluded that this screen and treat approach using HPV DNA testing identified and treated prevalent cases of CIN2+ and appeared to reduce the number of incident cases of CIN2+ that developed more than twelve months after cryotherapy.

Despite their many advantages, HPV screening tests (both standard and the rapid molecular tests) have a low positive predictive value for cervical cancer. They only indicate the presence of *current* HPV infection in a woman and cannot differentiate between women who simply have HPV infection (which might spontaneously clear) and those who have started to develop abnormal changes that might proceed to precancer and then cancer. Therefore, further follow-up testing would be warranted.

HPV Vaccine

Several HPV vaccines have been brought to market since 2006. Each is a preventive vaccine that works best before an individual is exposed to HPV (before the onset of sexual activity). The vaccine is considered to be the single most effective way to prevent cervical cancer. Three vaccines are approved by the FDA to prevent HPV infection: the quadrivalent HPV vaccine (Gardasil), which protects against four HPV types (6, 11, 16, and 18; HPV 6 and 11 cause 90 percent of genital warts); the bivalent HPV vaccine (Cervarix), which protects against two high-risk HPVs (16 and 18); and the nonavalent HPV vaccine (Gardasil 9), which prevents infection with the same four HPV types plus five additional high-risk HPV types (31, 33, 45, 52, and 58). (23–26) The vaccines are recommended for eleven- to twelve-year-old girls and boys, the age during which the immune response is high and exposure to the virus is low. The vaccine may be administered as young as age nine and until age twenty-six. Common side effects include pain and swelling at the site of injection.

Studies have shown that the HPV vaccine can prevent up to 66 to 96.6 percent of cervical cancers, depending on which HPV vaccine is used: bivalent, quadrivalent, or nonavalent. (27,28) Vaccines are given through a series of injections into muscle tissue over a six-month period. In 2016 the US Centers for Disease Control (CDC) changed its recommendation about the number of doses needed. The Advisory Committee on Immunization Practices for the CDC recommends that nine- to fourteen-year-olds need only two doses of the HPV vaccine, instead of the three doses that have traditionally been administered. The CDC determined that two doses within that age group are just as effective as three doses in older teens and young adults. (29) Since the HPV vaccine does not cover all the high-risk HPV types that cause cervical cancer, screening will be necessary even among those who receive the vaccine.

Recently the local Delhi government in India introduced an HPV vaccination program in public schools to include all nine- to thirteen-year-old girls. The Indian government received aid from the Global Alliance for Vaccines and Immunization (GAVI) to procure vaccines at a subsidized rate, which will make the HPV vaccine available for less than $5 a dose. The government also plans to expand the public-private partnership for cancer screening under the National Program for Prevention and Control of Cancer, Diabetes, Cardiovascular Diseases and Stroke (NPCDCS), to include cervical cancer screening. The NPCDCS program focuses on promotion of healthy lifestyles, early diagnosis and management of diabetes, hypertension, cardiovascular diseases, and common cancers (including cervical, breast, and oral). (30)

The development of safe and effective vaccines against HPV is acknowledged to be one of the more important breakthroughs in the fields of medicine and public health in the twenty-first century. The vaccine could have a major impact in India and other developing nations, given the high rate of undetected cervical cancer and the paucity of cervical cancer screening programs in those countries.

Program Challenges, Opportunities, and Possible Solutions: Education and Building Awareness

There is no doubt that globally we have attained significant milestones in detecting and treating early cervical changes by safe, simple, and inexpensive methods. However, implementing screening programs has not been easy. Finding the appropriate NGOs or institutions to partner with, recruiting the right staff to train, identifying appropriate training sites, and finding sufficient funding sources to ensure some degree of sustainability have individually and collectively been challenging. In addition, country partners have other competing needs, including managing public health programs such as sanitation, family planning, and chronic and acute disease prevention, which makes cervical cancer prevention less of a priority—not by will, but by necessity, mostly because of lack of awareness, funding, infrastructure, and human resources.

We often hear our partners state, "One of our main challenges is to find ways to motivate providers to offer cervical cancer preventive services, and to mobilize women to accept these services." It is well documented that education and information are basic factors that contribute to the success of an early diagnosis and treatment program. While many programs have created innovative materials that are culturally sensitive and linguistically appropriate, the ones that have the greatest impact, in our experience, are messages that are both inspirational and aspirational. That is, they motivate women to come forward on their own to get tested. The epic journey of Michele Baldwin (Lady Ganga) on the Ganges River is one such story.

Baldwin, a forty-three-year-old single mother of three, was told by her doctors that they could do nothing more to treat her cervical cancer. Baldwin decided to devote what time she had left to one extraordinary feat and disseminate a lifesaving message. She decided to take a trip to one of her favorite countries, India, and paddleboard 700 miles down the Ganges River to spread her message about the importance of cervical cancer screening. Her epic journey has been made into a short film and is in the process of being translated into several languages so that women around the world can be motivated and inspired to get screened for cervical cancer. We found that her film, *Lady Ganga, Nilza's Story*, puts to rest the questions, concerns, and excuses that so many women have: "Why should I get tested when I am feeling well?" "I do not want to show my pelvic area if I don't have to." "I have no one to take care of my young children." "I don't have transportation." "I cannot take time off from work." "I have to ask my husband first." We have found that women are receptive to inspirational educational messages, especially those presented in a manner that resonates personally. Stories like Baldwin's can have a tremendous impact on women of all ages.

More than 50 percent of India's population is below the age of forty. Harnessing the energy and enthusiasm of this cohort and providing these people with knowledge about cervical cancer could have a tremendous impact on reducing the burden of this disease. Our organization, in collaboration with one of our US partners, has developed a short, simple, and interactive presentation for middle and high school students. In this presentation the younger generation is encouraged to take a proactive role in getting vaccinated and to encourage their mothers, aunts, and older sisters to get screened. As Baldwin's eleven-year-old daughter eloquently said, "Doesn't matter if you don't know what a Pap is. Just ask your Mom if she got it."

While it is essential to provide education before screening, we have found that it is just as important to continue education after screening. Women who test negative should be told that while the negative test result is wonderful news, it is important to go for periodic screening. The absence of disease is not a guarantee that there is no disease, just as a positive test does not automatically mean that there is cancer. Educational campaigns should reinforce the message that women need to be screened periodically.

Screening and Treatment

"There are clinics that are offering cervical cancer screening without any clear pathway for follow-up and treatment," a program officer once said to me. Our belief is that there should be no screening unless a program is able to provide some accepted form of appropriate early treatment and a referral pathway for advanced cases wherever feasible. At one of our NGOs, where there were no doctors on-site and the community health workers were only trained in VIA and not in cryotherapy, the program coordinator conducted camps every four to six weeks and brought in doctors to treat the VIA positive cases.

The closer we get to one-stop screen and treat programs, the closer we are to reducing the number of late-stage cancers. Also, screening and treating at the same time has the potential to reduce the number of women lost to follow-up. It has also been our experience that when lunch and transportation are provided, attendance at screening camps improves, especially if women have to travel long distances.

Local community physicians and nurses would like to receive more support from the OB-GYN doctors. "Without their support, it is very difficult to scale up the VIA program," a community physician said. We at GIAHC are in complete agreement with this statement and believe that leadership from the OB-GYNs in the community plays an important and pivotal role in successful screening programs. These doctors can and should play a significant role in providing oversight and expertise.

In India the overwhelming majority of the population lives in rural settings, while the overwhelming majority of the physicians are located in urban centers. Most screening programs using VIA and cryotherapy are currently administered by OB-GYNs. By reorganizing the workforce, task shifting presents a viable solution for improving health care coverage, increasing capacity and making more efficient use of the human resources already available in areas where there is an acute shortage of doctors. We have worked with NGOs in very remote areas where there are no OB-GYNs.

We have trained the local midwives and Ayush doctors (doctors trained in Ayurvedic medicine, one of the oldest holistic healing systems) to screen for cervical cancer and provide the necessary education and information to the local community. If it were not for them, we would not have been able to carry out our work in such remote areas.

We have also found that partnering with medical institutions that have outreach programs is helpful. Some local community NGOs may not have the support of a network of physicians within their system. One NGO in a rural area of India stated the problem very eloquently: "We are trained in cryotherapy but have problems securing the tanks. Since we have no affiliation with the community OBGYNs or a nearby hospital where oxygen tanks and cryo tanks are supplied on a regular basis, we have no access to them. Besides, if we do not have affiliations, the OBGYNs and staff in the hospital double guess our work and compromise our image in our community."

In an effort to resolve the challenges of procuring cryotherapy tanks, we are now in the process of exploring newer devices that have been introduced in the market: CryoPens (using cold to freeze cells) and ThermoCoagulators (using heat to destroy abnormal tissue). Both devices are well suited for low resource settings, as they are inexpensive, portable, battery operated, and lightweight. A full charge is good for twenty-five to thirty treatments. The no-gas treatment options will substantially expand access to treatment through rural and mobile services.

One of our goals is to have the primary care staff in the rural areas be trained in VIA and cryotherapy and be able to refer advanced cases to local clinics where loop electrosurgical excision procedures (LEEP) can be performed. Some of our partners also have access to larger, tertiary centers with personnel who can manage the more advanced cases, including invasive cervical cancer.

"We are so glad that you asked us to present a clear pathway for treatment, referrals, budget, etc. as it forced us to review our capabilities and explore the facilities available in the neighboring areas to support our program. We just found out that there is an OB-GYN in the community who is very interested in cervical cancer prevention and has offered to help us with our referrals," one program manager told us.

Follow-up for Positive Cases

How a program handles the cases that are lost to follow-up is a crucial issue in the success of any cervical cancer screening program. A social worker told me, "Ma'am, when there is a VIA positive case, we do everything possible to make sure that the woman follows up for treatment. However, even knowing something could be wrong, many women refuse to come forward because they do not understand the disease process and its consequences. They talk to their friends and families, who discourage them to go for follow-up as they have no symptoms. So our program started a counseling service where women who tested positive attended the program and are grateful that they did as they are now cured of the disease." Counseling sessions and words of encouragement from doctors, nurses, and community advocates go a long way to help women make important decisions about their health.

Training

After our first foray in raising awareness and educating women about cervical cancer, we realized that there were very few programs offering cervical cancer education, screening, and early treatment training courses to physicians and nonphysicians in rural areas. When available, the programs were invariably in a different state where a different dialect was spoken, meaning that trainees would have to travel great distances, be away from home and work for several days, and face language barriers during training. This posed extra challenges to the learning process. In addition, we realized that many obstetrics residents were not trained in cryotherapy, and some were not familiar with LEEP. Discussions about offering a comprehensive cervical cancer prevention elective program to final year medical students ensued, as did holding periodic certification workshops for community doctors.

Our experience also taught us that practitioners who attended the training sessions had difficulty establishing cervical cancer screening programs. They had no idea where to begin or how to proceed. We also found that after providers are trained and return to their communities, there is very little ongoing support for them to initiate and sustain their programs. Some, feeling isolated and unsure of their skills, give up on the project.

In 2016 GIAHC accepted an invitation to participate in a partner workshop, Improving Data for Decision-Making in Global Cervical Cancer Programs (IDCCP), a project being led by the CDC, CDC Foundation, George W. Bush Institute, and WHO. Its objective is to develop a globally endorsed, standardized toolkit that can be adapted at the country level to support the collection of high-quality data for cervical cancer programs. The toolkit would also include a costing tool template that we believe would be a good starting point for programs that are interested in cervical cancer prevention.

Support Network for Community Health Centers

We have been exploring the feasibility of building capacity among community-based clinicians. One program that helps to foster such a relationship is Project ECHO (Extension for Community Healthcare Outcomes). Project ECHO links primary care clinicians with specialist care teams based at university medical centers to manage patients who have chronic conditions requiring complex care. It is transforming the way medical knowledge is shared and translated into everyday practice and, in the process, enabling thousands of people in remote and medically underserved communities to get care they couldn't easily get before, if at all. (31) Project ECHO has over ninety hubs worldwide—including more than fifty-five in the United States and more than thirty in sixteen additional countries—covering more than forty-five complex conditions. There are plans underway to develop an estimated fifty ECHO hubs or programs throughout India over the next four years to include management for various complex medical conditions, including cervical cancer.

Another challenge many cervical cancer screening programs face is personnel turnover, particularly among program coordinators. I once received a letter from a program coordinator stating, "Dear Dr. Krishnan. Thank you for giving me the opportunity to coordinate the cervical cancer prevention program. I have gained invaluable knowledge from this program. Based upon my experience, I have been offered a better job with better pay and benefits at a much bigger organization. I'm sorry that I have to leave, but as you will understand, I believe this is good for my career and future." While we are very happy for our staff to better their prospects, either through better jobs or receiving scholarships for higher education, it takes a long time to find adequate replacements, particularly in remote areas. Many programs are in danger of being completely derailed because of high turnover of trained staff. Other challenges that we continually encounter are in the area of financing. Fund-raising with matching programs and establishing corporate social responsibility (CSR)—a business approach that contributes to sustainable development by delivering economic, social, and environmental benefits for all stakeholders—have met with varying degrees of success. Often overlooked is the importance of maintaining a good database to monitor progress. Data are essential for many reasons, including program evaluation and presenting a rationale for funding.

Conclusion

Cervical cancer can have devastating effects on a woman and her family. This cancer in particular affects women in their prime. One out of every four cases of cervical cancer occurs in India, with a woman dying every seven to eight minutes from this disease. This situation can be explained by lack of access to effective screening and to services that facilitate early detection and treatment. As chapters in this book have shown, low-tech and inexpensive screening tools exist and could significantly reduce the burden of cervical cancer deaths, especially in less-developed countries. The sad thing is that cervical cancer is a disease that is almost completely preventable by vaccine and screening.

Our experience has shown that implementing a cervical cancer prevention program in India is challenging. There is a general lack of awareness among rural women, and finding appropriate partners can be difficult. In addition, insufficient funding from the government at the national level, lack of insurance coverage, lack of universal access to the HPV vaccine at affordable prices, and a fragmented health system make cervical cancer screening more challenging than it should be.

In spite of all these realities, there are many excellent cervical cancer prevention programs run by dedicated providers throughout the country. We are optimistic that with greater awareness of the need for screening, cervical cancer prevention will become routine and help substantially reduce the number of women who die from this disease. Michele Baldwin's quest, and her dying wish, was to spread the word about the importance of cervical cancer screening. We, and other organizations, are striving to ensure that women, especially poor, rural women, need not die of this preventable, treatable disease.

References

1. Lowy DR, Schiller JT. Reducing HPV-associated cancer globally. Cancer Prev Res (Phila) 2012;5(1):18–23.

2. Basic Information about HPV and cancer. Centers for Disease Control and Prevention; 2012/2013. Available from: https://www.cdc.gov/cancer/hpv/basic_info/.

3. Human papillomavirus (HPV) and cervical cancer. 2016. Available from: http://www.who.int/mediacentre/factsheets/fs380/en/.

4. WHO guidelines for screening and treatment of precancerous lesions for cervical cancer prevention. 2013. Available from: http://www.who.int/reproductivehealth/publications/cancers/screening_and_treatment_of_precancerous_lesions/en/.

5. Sankaranarayanan R, Budukh AM, Rajkumar R. Effective screening programmes for cervical cancer in low- and middle-income developing countries. Bull World Health Org 2001;79(10):954–62.

6. Consul S, Agrawal A, Sharma H, et al. Comparative study of effectiveness of Pap smear versus visual inspection with acetic acid and visual inspection with Lugol's iodine for mass screening of premalignant and malignant lesion of cervix. Indian J Med Paediatr Oncol 2012;33(3):161–5.

7. Carr KC, Sellors JW. Cervical cancer screening in low resource settings: using visual inspection with acetic acid. J Midwifery Womens Health 2004;49(4):329–37.

8. World Health Organization. Prevention of cervical cancer through screening using visual inspection with acetic acid (VIA) and treatment with cryotherapy: a demonstration project in six African countries: Malawi, Madagascar, Nigeria, Uganda, the United Republic of Tanzania, and Zambia. 2012. Available from: http://www.who.int/reproductivehealth/publications/cancers/9789241503860/en/.

9. Denny L, Quinn M, Sankaranarayanan R. Screening for cervical cancer in developing countries. Sci Dir Vaccine 2006;24S3:S3/71–7.

10. Khan MJ, Mark S, Jose J. Accuracy of human papillomavirus testing in primary screening of cervical neoplasia: results from a multicenter study in India. Int J Cancer 2005;(116):230–1.

11. Sankaranarayanan R, Basu P, Wesley RS, et al. Accuracy of visual screening for cervical neoplasia: results from an IARC multicentre study in India and Africa. Int J Cancer 2004;110:907–13.

12. Sankaranarayanan R, Esmy PO, Rajkumar R, et al. Effect of visual screening on cervical cancer incidence and mortality in Tamil Nadu, India: a cluster-randomised trial. Lancet 2007;370:398–406.

13. Nieminen P, Vuorma S, Viikki M, et al. Comparison of HPV test versus conventional and automation-assisted Pap screening as potential screening tools for preventing cervical cancer. BJOG 2004;111(8):842–8.

14. Sankaranarayanan R, Gaffikin L, Jacob M, Robles S. A critical assessment of screening methods for cervical neoplasia. Int J Gynecol Obstet 2005;89(Suppl 2): S4–12.

15. Dillner J. Primary human papillomavirus testing in organized cervical screening. Curr Opin Obstet Gynecol 2013;25(1):11–6.

16. Ogilvie GS, Patrick DM, Schulzer M, et al. Diagnostic accuracy of self-collected vaginal specimens for human papillomavirus compared to clinician collected human papillomavirus specimens: a meta-analysis. Sex Transm Infect 2005;81:207–12.

17. Snijders PJ, Verhoef VM, Arbyn M, et al. High-risk HPV testing on self-sampled versus clinician-collected specimens: a review on the clinical accuracy and impact on population attendance in cervical cancer screening. Int J Cancer 2013;132:2223–36.

18. Untiet S, Vassilakos P, McCarey C, et al. HPV self-sampling as primary

screening test in sub-Saharan Africa: implication for a triaging strategy. Int J Cancer 2014;135:1911–7.

19. Lazcano-Ponce E, Lorincz AT, Cruz-Valdez A, et al. Self-collection of vaginal specimens for human papillomavirus testing in cervical cancer prevention (MARCH): a community-based randomised controlled trial. Lancet 2011;378:1868–73.

20. Ying H, Jing F, Fanghui Z, et al. High-risk HPV nucleic acid detection kit—the careHPV test—a new detection method for screening. Sci Rep 2014;4. doi: 10.1038/srep04704.

21. Shi J, Canfell K, Lew JB, et al. Evaluation of primary HPV-DNA testing in relation to visual inspection methods for cervical cancer screening in rural China: an epidemiologic and cost-effectiveness modelling study. BMC Cancer 2011;11:239. doi: 10.1186/1471-2407-11-239.

22. Denny L, Kuhn L, Hu CC, et al. Human papillomavirus-based cervical cancer prevention: long-term results of a randomized screening trial. J Natl Cancer Inst 2010;102:157–67.

23. Schiller JT, Castellsague X, Garland SM. A review of clinical trials of human papillomavirus prophylactic vaccines. Vaccine 2012;30(Suppl 5):F123–38.

24. Kjær SK, Sigurdsson K, Iversen OE, et al. A pooled analysis of continued prophylactic efficacy of quadrivalent human papillomavirus (Types 6/11/16/18) vaccine against high-grade cervical and external genital lesions. Cancer Prev Res 2009;2:868–78.

25. The FUTURE II Study Group. Quadrivalent vaccine against human papillomavirus to prevent high-grade cervical lesions. N Engl J Med 2007;356:1915–27.

26. Chatterjee A. The next generation of HPV vaccines: nonavalent vaccine V503 on the horizon. Expert Rev Vaccines 2014;13(11):1279–90.

27. Jit M, Brisson M, Laprise, J, Choi YH. Comparison of two doses and three doses of human papillomavirus vaccine schedules: cost effectiveness analysis based on transmission model. BMJ 2015;350:g7584.

28. Gee J, Naleway A, Shui I, et al. Monitoring the safety of quadrivalent human papillomavirus vaccine: findings from the Vaccine Safety Datalink. Vaccine 2011;29(46):8279–84.

29. CDC announces changes to HPV vaccine dose recommendation. 2016 Oct 24. Available from: http://www.capradio.org/articles/2016/10/24/cdc-announces-changes-to-hpv-vaccine-dose-recommendation/.

30. National Programme for Prevention and Control of Cancer, Diabetes, Cardiovascular Diseases and Stroke (NPCDCS). Available from: http://www.nrhmhp.gov.in/sites/default/files/files/NCD_Guidelines.pdf.

31. Project ECHO. Available from: http://echo.unm.edu/.

Chapter 4

Biswajit Paul and Rita Isaac

Educate, Screen, and Treat Program for Cervical Cancer in Rural Tamil Nadu, India

Mariamma's Story

ariamma is a forty-year-old married woman with two children who lost her husband to a traffic accident. She has a son who had twelve years of schooling and is working as a daily laborer. Her daughter passed her twelfth standard examination and aspires to become a nurse. At present Mariamma works as a daily laborer in a government-sponsored work program. She is satisfied with her life and is thankful to God to be alive and healthy and in a position to help her family.

Mariamma's story could have been much different had she not visited one of the cervical cancer screening camps conducted by Rural Unit for Health and Social Affairs (RUHSA) Department of the Christian Medical College (CMC), Vellore, in the state of Tamil Nadu (TN), India. She came to know about the cervical cancer screening program for women from the health education sessions given by RUHSA public health nurses and health workers. One day she decided to visit one such clinic, which was being held in a neighboring village, for a checkup. Although she did not have any symptoms related to the reproductive tract, she decided to give it a try, as the health workers had said repeatedly that a routine checkup at least once is helpful. In the health camp, she saw other women from her village who had come for cervical cancer screening.

The screening program was much more than a quick exam. The women were told about woman's reproductive health, symptoms related to cervical cancer, and the benefits of undergoing the screening. After giving her consent, Mariamma was examined and screened in a separate room using the visual inspection with acetic acid (VIA) method. This is an excellent test to use in rural areas. It is a quick test, not expensive at all; results are immediate; and it is not painful or very uncomfortable. Mariamma was told that she had a positive VIA screen and that she should go to the RUHSA outpatient clinic for confirmation and discussion of treatment options. Naturally she was shocked and scared. At RUHSA a biopsy was taken and sent to the tertiary hospital in Vellore. The pathology report showed squamous cell carcinoma. When this news was broken to her, she cried inconsolably; she thought she was going to die. Her thoughts immediately went to her children: What would happen to her children should she die? After she was told that her condition was treatable, she was reassured and began treatment at the Christian Medical College (CMC) in Vellore. She underwent surgery, during which her uterus and right ovary and fallopian tube were removed, and her bilateral pelvic lymph nodes were resected. The follow-up histological report on the tissues showed it to be cervical intraepithelial neoplasia 3 (CIN3). CIN is divided into grades, which describe how far the abnormal cells have gone into the surface layer of the cervix. CIN3 indicates abnormal changes (but not cancer) affecting the full thickness of the surface layer of the cervix. After Mariamma was discharged, home visits by RUHSA health workers were scheduled. Fortunately, Mariamma recovered fully. After three months' rest she returned to work and now continues to work to support her family.

This story could have had a very different ending had Mariamma not taken part in the cervical cancer screening program. In her own words, "I got my life because of RUHSA and thank you for everything that you have done. I can't describe in words how grateful I am to you." She strongly believes in the cervical cancer screening program and says that it is lifesaving. She now recommends screening to her female friends, relatives, and neighbors and asks them to get it done if they are between thirty and fifty years of age.

Cervical Cancer in India: The Backdrop

Cervical cancer is one of the most common cancers affecting women worldwide, although the overwhelming majority of cases occur in the developing countries. Most of the cases of death are also reported from the developing world, where the disease is often detected late and treatment options are limited. Late detection of the disease calls for more radical treatment that involves more costs and greater suffering on the part of the patient and her family; often families are not able to afford treatment and go through great agony. A major problem in rural areas and in developing countries is the lack of trained personnel available to provide screening and subsequent treatment. Often health facilities and health personnel are not available, especially for rural, poor women.

Cervical cancer affects not only the individual woman but also the entire family and community. In Mariamma's case, had her cancer not been detected, in all likelihood she would have died, thus orphaning her children. Decisions on how best to use scarce resources to diagnose and treat cervical precancer must consider the extent of disability and death caused by the disease and the likely success of an intervention to reduce the suffering and death associated with that disease versus using scarce resources to prevent or control other illnesses. (1) Cervical cancer, when seen through this lens, can cause a high burden of disability and death; the intervention (screening and treatment of precancer) can mitigate the effect of the disease to a large extent. This makes cervical cancer prevention and control a rational and ethical imperative.

Worldwide, each year 528,000 cases of cervical cancer are detected and 266,000 women die of this disease; it is the fourth most common cancer among women. About 85 percent of all cases of cervical cancer are reported from developing countries, where it accounts for 12 percent of all female cancers. (2,3) Almost half of the cervical cancer cases occur in women younger than fifty years of age, (4) and women with only a primary-level education or who are illiterate are seven times more likely to develop cervical cancer than those with a secondary-level education. It also has been shown that rural women have poorer survival rates than their urban counterparts. (5–9) India contributes one-fifth of all cases of cervical cancer and one-quarter of all deaths due to cervical cancer worldwide, and the disease is the second most common cancer among women in India. (2) As of 2012, more than 67,000 deaths occur in India every year, with an age-standardized incidence rate of 22 per 100,000 women and an age-standardized mortality rate of 12.4 per 100,000 women. (10,11)

The precipitating cause of cervical cancer is well defined. Infections with human papillomavirus (HPV) are responsible for virtually all cases of cervical cancer. Cervical precancer and cancer are primarily seen in those who have persistent or chronic infections with one or more of the oncogenic variants of HPV. Women living with HIV/AIDS are more likely to develop persistent HPV infections, which lead to cervical cancer, at an earlier age. (12) Screening is a powerful tool to target the cervical precancer stage and allow for timely intervention. The ten- to twenty-year lag period between precancer and cancer provides an opportunity to screen, detect, and treat precancer and prevent its progression to cancer. Several screening tests are available that effectively detect precancer, and there are also several afford-able treatment options.

The Papanicolaou (Pap) test has been used as the gold standard screening test for cervical carcinoma and has been effective in reducing the incidence of and mortality from the disease. It is a highly specific test, on the order of 95 to 99 percent specificity (13–15); however, the sensitivity ranges between 60 and 90 percent. (16–17) One of the drawbacks to this screening method is that it requires highly trained human resources, including a cytology lab with trained cytologists, a substantial amount of laboratory equipment, and multiple hospital visits by the patient. Patients must wait days, in some cases weeks, for lab results, and follow-up can be difficult if the patient lives far from the clinic or hospital.

Pap screening programs are standard in the developed world, but in much of the developing world, especially rural areas, such a test is imprac-tical and usually impossible to do. Most developing countries have a poor health infrastructure, limited financial capabilities, and a small human resource pool, as well as a sociocultural milieu and an understanding of the disease that differ from those in more developed countries. Therefore the approach to screening for cervical cancer needs to be tailored to the location.

What could be used in lieu of the Pap test? There is a need for alternate screening tests in rural areas that would be sufficiently sensitive and spe-cific, be easy to administer, not rely on cytology, be cost efficient, not require much expertise, and provide quick results. The tests developed include the VIA, visual inspection with Lugol's iodine (VILI), and human papillomavi-rus (HPV) testing. Each test has its strengths and weaknesses. In addition, a more high-tech test, molecular HPV testing, is based on the detection of DNA from high-risk HPV types in vaginal and/or cervical samples (an ex-ample is the hybrid capture 2 test). Testing is done on women under thirty years of age. However, this test is much more expensive than the VIA or VILI tests, and a positive result in a woman over the age of thirty indicates that she *may* have an existing lesion or *may* be at risk for future precancer and cancer. An HPV test only confirms that a woman has an infection; it does not confirm that the woman has precancer. Women who test positive for HPV have be to further screened with cytology or VIA to confirm a lesion. Logistics, costs, and patient refusal of additional treatment are common barriers to providing the necessary care to women who test positive. We have seen this to be true in our program.

Several studies have found VIA to be a suitable alternative to cytology as a population-based screening test, especially in low-resource settings. The sensitivity of VIA ranges between 66 and 96 percent (median 84%) and the specificity between 64 and 98 percent (median 82%); the positive predictive value ranges from 10 to 20 percent and the negative predictive value from 92 to 97 percent. (18–24) In studies in which VIA was compared to cytology in the same setting, VIA performed similarly to (and sometimes better than) cytology in terms of detecting high-grade lesions or cancer, but was less specific. (25) The addition of magnification to VIA (VIAM) does not seem to improve the accuracy of the test. (18)

An alternate strategy created by the World Health Organization (WHO) for developing countries is the "screen and treat" approach, in which the treatment decision is based on a screening test, not on a histologically confirmed diagnosis. (26) (See figure 4.1.) Treatment, which is provided immediately or soon after a positive screening test result, includes cryotherapy and loop electrosurgical excision procedure (LEEP). Women who test positive undergo a biopsy and then, if warranted, have cryotherapy or LEEP performed. Cervical cancer screening should be performed at least once for every woman between thirty and forty-nine years of age, although evidence suggests that even being screened only once in a lifetime is beneficial. Ideally, women who test negative for VIA or cytology should be rescreened every three to five years. Women who test negative for HPV testing are rescreened every five years. (27–28)

The RUHSA Educate, Screen, and Treat Program: A Model Example of Screening in Resource-Poor Areas

The Rural Unit of Health and Social Affairs (RUHSA) provides primary- and secondary-level health care to the rural population through a seventy-bed hospital and eighteen outreach clinics across the K. V. Kuppam community development block (clinic catchment area), one of the large southern states of India. It is located approximately 130 kilometers from Chennai, the capital city of Tamil Nadu, and covers a population of 138,803. The area is

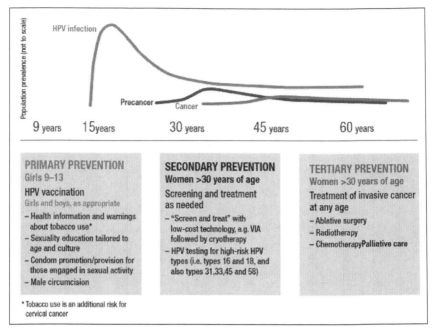

Figure 4.1. The WHO comprehensive approach to cervical cancer prevention and control: overview of programmatic interventions over the life course to prevent HPV infection and cervical cancer. Source: WHO guidance note: comprehensive cervical cancer prevention and control: a healthier future for girls and women. Geneva: World Health Organization; 2013.

characterized as rural, with a population predominantly of low to middle socioeconomic status. Most of the population is agrarian; men work as laborers in the fields. Women mostly stay at home and take care of the family; the literacy rate among women is 57 percent, and many of the women have fewer than ten years of schooling. There are not many job opportunities for youths, who have started going to neighboring cities to work in large factories or manufacturing units. Health care is provided through rural clinics similar to RUHSA.

RUHSA treats about 10,000 patients per month from K. V. Kuppam and neighboring blocks. The main hospital in Vellore provides specialist outpatient and inpatient care in pediatrics, obstetrics and gynecology, ophthalmology, otorhinolaryngology, orthopedics, and surgery. RUHSA also runs specialized clinics for the local community, including a diabetic clinic, an elderly clinic, a mental health clinic, and an infectious disease (ID) clinic. RUHSA provides primary care through its outreach clinics, including treatment for common illnesses, chronic disease management, and antenatal care. A health team that includes a doctor, a public health nurse, a rural community officer, health aides, and family care volunteers provides primary care at the community level through these outreach clinics. The Christian Medical College and Hospital, located 25 kilometers away at Vellore Town, serves as a referral center for patients requiring more complicated care and follow-up.

In 1997 India launched a national program, Reproductive and Child Health Program (RCH), to strengthen women's and children's health. One of the components of the program is prevention of reproductive tract infections (RTIs) and sexually transmitted infections (STIs). RUHSA already had a strong maternal and child health component from its beginning, and this was expanded in 1997 to include RTI/STI. It became apparent that the incidence and prevalence of cervical cancer were high. Advanced stages were commonly seen. The women had neither the knowledge about the disease nor the opportunity for early treatment. Most, if not all, rural clinics did not screen for this disease.

In 2007 RUHSA launched its educate, screen, and treat program for cervical cancer with the aim of early detection, treatment, and education. The program combined health literacy with community outreach screening by public health nurses to address the high incidence of cervical cancer in rural Tamil Nadu. The program has been integrated into primary care through these outreach clinics to improve acceptance among the local community.

The Process

One of the essential activities of the program is to screen women between the ages of thirty and fifty using VIA as the screening modality. Women are encouraged to participate in the screening program by peers who have been screened (peer self-help educators), as well as by community public health educators. An important component of the program is having public health nurses spread the message during their visits to the community.

Screening is done at the eighteen outreach clinics, which also provide general medical care and antenatal care for women. Each room is well equipped with a light source and a trolley containing instruments, swabs and other materials required for screening. Freshly prepared 5 percent acetic acid solution is used for painting the cervix, and naked eye observations are made to detect VIA positive cases. All these processes are done by the public health nurses, who are well trained in doing speculum examination and VIA testing and interpretation. A separate room enables health care providers to speak privately with the patient before and after the screening test.

All women who test positive for VIA are referred to the secondary-level community health center at RUHSA, where a second VIA test is done to confirm the findings. Cryotherapy can be done at RUHSA; however, women who require more advanced care are referred to Christian Medical College and Hospital in Vellore Town for further management. Patients treated with cryotherapy are asked to come for follow-up at RUHSA, and cases treated at the tertiary hospital are also followed up monthly at the oncology clinic at RUHSA.

Health Education and Awareness

Health education and awareness are important and integral components of the screening program. In addition to providing information, RUHSA also presents classes on empowerment to help women make informed decisions about their health as well as that of their family. There has been a systematic effort to educate the women in the RUHSA catchment area as well as to involve the men and village leaders. Without "buy in" from the local women, the male village leaders, and the local community in general, our program would not be as successful as it is.

Since screening was a new concept to the residents of the rural blocks, and since it involved women coming for examination when they were apparently healthy or asymptomatic, a lot of effort was initially put in to help the women understand the need for screening and understand and accept its potential benefits, as well as to encourage them to come to be screened. We approached this task by providing community education through well-organized self-help groups of women who were trained to act as peer educators for women in the community. These self-help groups were established through micro-finance schemes and income-generation initiatives for women; the women selected were proactive, respected members of their local communities. This strategy helped to make the screening program more acceptable, as these were local women whom the community knew and trusted.

During 2009, women group leaders were selected and trained as peer educators by the RUHSA team. These training sessions were intensive and designed to educate the women about signs and symptoms of cervical cancer and its causes, the benefits of screening, and the treatment modalities available. It was stressed that screening was a simple, painless procedure. During this four-month period, sixteen educational programs were conducted, and we trained approximately 1,000 self-help group members.

We recognized that involving the male members of the community and gaining their trust was also important for the screening program to gain momentum. The sociocultural milieu of the rural Indian community is such that the husbands' consent plays an important role in the life of the women. The RUHSA team organized meetings with local male government leaders and other key male members of the village community and informed them about the screening program and its benefits. These activities were supplemented by integrating a cervical cancer community education program into RUHSA's routine evening health education program using hand-puppet audiovisual shows. Educational materials like flip charts, posters, banners, and drawings were developed for visual appreciation and understanding; these were tailor-made taking into account the local cultural norms and rural background.

Sustained effort was necessary, and newer techniques were introduced periodically. One of the interventions aimed at increasing the knowledge and acceptance of cervical cancer screening was using mobile health (mHealth) technology. Mobile phones were used to communicate with rural women using an integrated voice response system (IVRS) to tell them about cervical carcinoma through frequently asked questions (FAQ) and to address doubts and answer questions posted by the women. This helped in empowering women to make their own decisions on screening and treatment for cervical cancer rather than being dependent on their husbands or public health workers. mHealth was also used in this program for monitoring and follow-up of VIA positive cases. There is a concerted, continuous effort to integrate cervical cancer screening into routine practice in the lives of the rural Indian women, similar to the process we adopted for routine immunization.

Training

As a part of the educate, screen, and treat program for cervical carcinoma, training was also organized periodically for groups and local individual health practitioners who were involved in patient care and were interested in starting their own cervical cancer screening programs in their practices. Over the course of four years, RUHSA held several three-day workshops

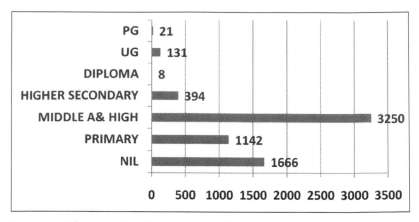

Figure 4.2. Educational levels of patients with invasive cervical cancer

for the local practitioners. Participants included both doctors and nurses. Intensive hands-on training was given on VIA, colposcopy, and cryotherapy, along with a few theoretical sessions on cervical cancer. The hands-on training sessions were held at RUHSA and also in the primary care outreach clinics in the community; this was to give the participants a sense of how a screening program can be set up and practiced in the community. A few medical schools and secondary-level mission hospitals with community outreach facilities have become our partners in this program and have successfully implemented the cervical cancer screening program in their local communities.

Outcome: Did These Efforts Bear Fruit?

Over ten years 6,612 local women were screened by RUHSA, with 80 VIA positive cases being detected and 137 cases of invasive cervical cancer being diagnosed. (5) The educational level of the women is presented in figure 4.2. Treatment with cryotherapy was possible in 29 of the VIA positive cases. Biopsies were done in 32 cases, of which 11 were CIN1, 2 were CIN2, and 3 were CIN3. Biopsies were sent to CMC, Vellore, and staging was done. The higher-grade cancers were treated with various treatment modalities, such as radical surgery, chemotherapy, radiotherapy, or a combination of these. Most of the cases of invasive cancer were found to be in stages IIIB, IIB, and IB, in that order.

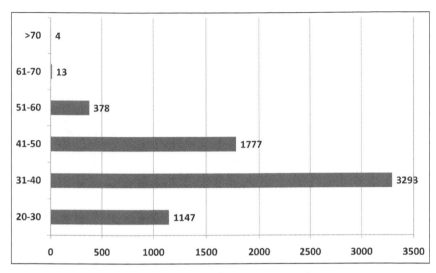

Figure 4.3. Age distribution of patients with invasive cervical cancer

The age distribution of the women screened for cervical carcinoma in the last ten years is shown in figure 4.3. The peak incidence of invasive cervical carcinoma was in the thirty- to fifty-year-old group (58.4%). However, recently there has been a decrease in the invasive cancers being picked up by the program, with smaller numbers of higher-stage cancers being reported. The stage IV and stage III invasive cancers have declined considerably since 2010, and stage I and stage II cancers are more commonly detected; in fact, there were no cases of stage IV.

Active follow-up with patients was started recently to provide information about the status of patients with invasive cervical cancer who were diagnosed at RUHSA and referred to the tertiary center for treatment. Follow-up was done through visits to the community that served to motivate patients to visit the monthly oncology clinic run at RUHSA. What we found out came as a big revelation to us and was an important milestone in the learning curve of understanding the human behavioral patterns in the context of the screening program. Data showed 49 deaths (40.2%) among 122 patients diagnosed with invasive cancer in the pre-follow-up period. The data indicate that without proper follow-up and support for patients after the diagnosis, lives will be lost. Assistance is important to help patients get appointments at tertiary care centers.

Table 4.1. Follow-up on Invasive Cancer Patients

	Until 2014 (before follow-up)		2015 Onward (after follow-up)	
Treatment method	Cases	Deaths	Cases	Deaths
RT and chemotherapy at CMC	43	11	11	1
Treatment not taken	25	21	1	1
Government hospital treated	23	16	5	1
Surgery	1	0	0	0
Not available	30	1	0	0
TOTAL	122	49	17	3

Table 4.1 illustrates the results for the invasive cancer patients, dividing them into pre- and post-follow-up periods. When follow-up was started in 2015 and we began to collect data on all patients who had been diagnosed with cervical cancer at RUHSA, we found that it took quite some time for patients to agree to get treatment. Many (20.5%) did not seek treatment at all, and 30 (24.6%) were lost to follow-up. The post-follow-up period was much better, with almost all patients taking treatment (94%), fewer deaths (17.6%), and no loss to follow-up. Regular follow-up and support can play a vital role in saving lives and is an essential part of any successful screening program.

The Challenges

As the program has evolved, we found that lack of awareness about cervical cancer is one of the major challenges that we need to address more closely. (29) Before our program, the overwhelming majority of the village women did not know about cervical cancer. They did not know what the signs and symptoms of the disease were. They were not aware that it is the most common cancer among rural Indian women and that they are at highest risk for the disease because of their low socioeconomic status and low educational level. Lack of awareness about the disease, its manifestations, the course of illness, and availability of screening and treatment modalities were some issues that had to be addressed time and again to instill a sense of goodwill and ownership toward the program. It was challenging to convince the local women that the program was about a disease that is prevalent but shows no symptoms in the early stages. It can be treated successfully if diagnosed at an early stage.

Even ten years into the program, some women are still ignorant about the disease. It is clear to us that continuous education and publicity about the program are necessary. One of the learning points from the program was how to think like the people in the community so as to design a health message that would be not only relevant but also acceptable to them. Thinking like an expert does not always work. Because cervical cancer screening involves an invasive examination of genitalia and because of the stigma of having a "sexual" disease, the educational message of our cervical cancer program had to be tailored to address the fears, myths, and misconceptions of the local population. We found out that we had touched on a sensitive issue and a socioculturally unacceptable norm of their lives. For a woman, coming to a screening camp for cervical cancer is like posting an advertisement in the community about her health, her sexual being. In addition, the mention of the word "cancer" frightened the women. So we did a course correction and instead of "cancer camps" we held "health camps" and integrated cervical cancer screening with eye screening and dental health screening. Through the outreach clinics we folded the entire cancer screening program into primary health care, which also had a component of women's health check-up, including screening by VIA. This proved to be a brilliant move on our part, and acceptance of the program increased substantially.

Another challenge to the educate, screen, and treat program was convincing women to come for screening. When we would talk about it in a closed group or meetings, some woman would ask: "Why should I come to hospital for a test when I am well?" The concept of screening is unknown in rural Indian populations; the local women had never thought of it and were not convinced that it was worthwhile to spend their time and money on it. It took time to convince them that screening for cervical cancer really helps and can even save their lives. The success stories of other women in the community who had come for screening have really helped. Each woman coming for screening or getting treatment increased community confidence. We hope a time will come when women will not think twice about the benefits of screening, just as they do not think twice when they bring their babies to the clinic for vaccination.

With all the efforts to make the screening program a success and establish a routine for cervical cancer screening among women thirty to fifty years of age, financial constraints remain a major problem. After being diagnosed for cervical cancer, getting treatment can be a long and costly process. Health insurance is unheard of in this part of the world, and spending out-of-pocket is not possible given the local people's meager incomes. Only a few government centers are available for treatment, and large corporate, private hospitals are out of financial reach for these patients. CMC Vellore is a not-for-profit organization that as part of its mission does help some patients who are in dire financial situations. Treating departments sometimes write off the charges, but this is a stopgap measure that over the long term is probably not sustainable. So the major issue is how to generate funds and set aside a corpus for patients whereby treatment can be facilitated. There is also an urgent need for political will and government planning and financing to make it a sustainable program for the masses, taking into account the sheer numbers of patients that screening would generate.

Hopes for the Future

Amid all the challenges and obstacles that we have had to deal with, new horizons and hope always exist. Where we found the challenge of lack of awareness and education in the rural community, we also found newer methods of health education and galvanized support of female self-help groups to spread the word on screening and treatment of cervical cancer. Local community members and female group leaders became agents of change and helped to strengthen the program. We realized that we should use the community as a resource and the capabilities of the community for the benefit of the community.

Mobile technology can provide a great opportunity for relating with people, be it for delivering health messages, following up and monitoring, or keeping tabs on an individual patient's progress. mHealth and eHealth are great tools to take any program forward. We hope that in the near future they will open up a world of opportunities that can improve health care delivery in rural India. It is often said that in India there are more mobile phones than toilets! We have capitalized on this to our advantage.

Indian state and local governments have started to become more involved in cancer screening programs. Although this is only the first step, it gives us hope that in future the treatment costs for patients can be taken care of by multiple means of financing. The present Indian government has started a cancer screening program for cervical, oral, and breast cancer and aims to establish such programs in one hundred districts in the first phase; this will be population-based screening targeting the rural, poor vulnerable population over thirty years of age. The screening will be free of cost, and the detected cancer cases will be treated in the community health centers, district hospitals, and tertiary hospitals run by government, wherever the most appropriate treatment options are available. As a part of the program, the government also aims at providing some cancer drugs free of cost to patients. (30,31) Another optimistic course of action taken by the present government is the founding of health insurance schemes covering the poor and the marginalized that will help in reducing a part of the burden of health care.

The fight against cervical cancer has to be fought on many fronts. Primary, secondary, and tertiary levels of prevention have to be applied if we are to succeed in our mission to significantly reduce the mortality and morbidity from cervical cancer. Two important goals for RUHSA in primary prevention are health education and HPV vaccination. Health education should be provided to adolescents and adults, in schools and in community education programs, individually as well as in appropriate groups; it includes education on sexuality, reproductive hygiene, and the use of condoms and should encompass social and cultural norms of the community. HPV vaccination should be given to girls under fifteen years of age or per the national program. Secondary prevention should include screening of all women between thirty and fifty years of age with any of the methods mentioned above. The goal of tertiary prevention is to prevent deaths due to cervical cancer and includes treatment of invasive cancer with modalities appropriate for its stage as well as palliative care to relieve pain and suffering.

Mariamma was only one of the many women who have benefited from our cervical cancer screening program. Many more are taking advantage of screening, not only for themselves, but also for their families. The communities in our health care catchment area have come to realize that screening can save lives. It took many years to achieve this acceptance and trust, but the end results show that it was well worth the wait.

References

1. Comprehensive cervical cancer control: a guide to essential practice. 2nd ed. Geneva: World Health Organization; 2014.

2. World Health Organization. International Agency for Research on Cancer. GLOBOCON 2012: estimated cancer incidence, mortality, and prevalence worldwide in 2012. Available from: http://globocan.iarc.fr/old/FactSheets/cancers/cervix-new.asp.

3. Cervical cancer screening in developing countries: report of a WHO consultation. World Health Organization; 2002. Available from: http://apps.who.int/iris/bitstream/10665/42544/1/9241545720.pdf.

4. Chhabra S, Bhavani M, Mahajan N, Bawaskar R. Cervical cancer in Indian rural women: trends over two decades. J Obstet Gynaecol 2010;30:725–8.

5. Isaac R, Finkel M, Olver I, et al. Translating evidence into practice in low resource settings: cervical cancer screening tests are only part of the solution in rural India. Asian Pac J Cancer Prev 2012;13: 4169–72.

6. Dinshaw K, Mishra G, Shastri S, et al. Determinants of compliance in a cluster randomised controlled trial on screening of breast and cervix cancer in Mumbai. Oncol 2007;73:3–4.

7. Kaku M, Mathew A, Rajan B. Impact of socio-economic factors in delayed reporting and late-stage presentation among patients with cervix cancer in a major cancer hospital in South India. Asian Pac J Cancer Prev 2008;9:589–94.

8. Nandakumar A, Anantha N, Venugopal TC. Incidence, mortality and survival in cancer of the cervix in Bangalore, India. Brit J Cancer 1995;71:1348–52.

9. Swaminathan R, Selvakumaran R, Esmy PO, et al. Cancer pattern and survival in a rural district in South India. Cancer Epidemiol, 2009;33:325–31.

10. Sreedevi A, Javed R, Dinesh A. Epidemiology of cervical cancer with special focus on India. Int J Womens Health 2015;7:405–14.

11. Bruni L, Barrionuevo-Rosas L, Albero G, et al. ICO Information Centre on HPV and Cancer (HPV Information Centre). Human papillomavirus and related diseases in India. Summary Report. 2017. Available from: http://www.hpvcentre.net/statistics/reports/XWX.pdf.

12. WHO guidance note: comprehensive cervical cancer prevention and control: a healthier future for girls and women. Geneva: WHO; 2013. Available from: http://www.who.int/reproductivehealth/publications/cancers/9789241505147/en/.

13. Agency for Health Care Policy and Research. Evaluation of cervical cytology. Technology Assessment Report No. 5. Rockville, MD: Agency for Health Care Policy and Research; 1999. Available from: http://www.ahcpr.gov.

14. Fahey MT, Irwig L, Macaskill P. Meta-analysis of Pap test accuracy. Am J Epidemiol 1995;141:680–9.

15. Nanda K, McCrory DC, Myers ER, et al. Accuracy of the Papanicolau test in

screening for and follow-up of cervical cytologic abnormalities: a systematic review. Ann Intern Med 2000;132:810–9.

16. Boyes DA, Morrison B, Knox Eg, Miller A. A cohort study of cervical cancer screening in British Columbia. Clin Invest Med 1982;5:1–29.

17. IARC Working Group on Cervical Cancer Screening. In: Hakama M, Miller AB, Day NE, editors. Screening for cancer of the uterine cervix. IARC Scientific Publications No. 76. Lyon: International Agency for Research on Cancer; 1986. p. 133–42.

18. Frisch LE, Milner FH, Ferris DG. Naked-eye inspection of the cervix after acetic acid application may improve the predictive value of negative cytologic screening. J Fam Pract 1994;39:457–60.

19. Cecchini S, Bonardi R, Mazzotta A, et al. Testing cervicography and VIA as screening tests for cervical cancer. Tumori 1993;79:22–5.

20. Megavand E, Denny L, Dehaeck K, et al. Acetic acid visualization of the cervix: an alternative to cytologic screening. Obstet Gynecol 1996;88:383–6.

21. Denny L, Kuhn L, Pollack A, et al. Evaluation of alternative methods of cervical cancer screening for resource-poor settings. Cancer 2000;89:826–33.

22. Londhe M, George SS, Seshadri L. Detection of CIN by naked eye visualization after application of acetic acid. Indian J Cancer 1997;34:88–91.

23. Sankaranarayanan R, Gaffikin L, Jacob M, et al. A critical assessment of screening methods for cervical neoplasia. Int J Gynaecol Obstet 2005;89(Suppl 2):S4–12.

24. Gaffikin L, McGrath JA, Arbyn M, Blumenthal PD. Visual inspection with acetic acid as a cervical cancer test: accuracy validated using latent class analysis. BMC Med Res Methodol 2007;7:36.

25. University of Zimbabwe/JHPIEGO Cervical Cancer Project. Visual inspection with acetic acid for cervical cancer screening: test qualities in a primary-care setting. Lancet 1999;353:869–73.

26. WHO guidelines for screening and treatment of precancerous lesions for cervical cancer prevention. Geneva: WHO; 2013. Available from: http://www.who.int/reproductivehealth/publications/cancers/screening_and_treatment_of_precancerous_lesions/en/.

27. WHO guidelines: treatment of cervical intraepithelial neoplasia 2–3 and adenocarcinoma in situ. Geneva: WHO; 2014. Available from: http://www.who.int/reproductivehealth/publications/cancers/treatment_CIN_2-3/en/)

28. WHO guidelines: use of cryotherapy for cervical intraepithelial neoplasia. Geneva: WHO; 2011. Available from: http://www.who.int/reproductivehealth/publications/cancers/9789241502856/en/.

29. Isaac, R, Finkel, ML, Trevena, L, et al. An educational training cervical cancer screening program for rural health care providers in India. Indian J Community Health 2014;26:115–8.

30. Soon, cancer screening centres in 100 districts across India. The Indian Express

2016 Jun 21. Available from: http://indianexpress.com/article/lifestyle/health/health-ministry-soon-cancer-screening-centres-in-100-districts-2865536/.

31. Govt. to make screening of oral, cervix, and breast cancer mandatory for 30+ from November 2016. The India Today 2016 Oct 10. Available from: http://india today.intoday.in/story/govt-to-make-screening-of-oral-cervix-and-breast-cancer-mandatory-for-30-from-november-2016/1/783976.html.

Chapter 5

Christine Campbell and Heather A. Cubie

Delivering a Screen and Treat Program in Rural Malawi

The Nkhoma Story

Malawi is a small, landlocked country in sub-Saharan eastern Africa with a population of 17.2 million (as of 2015). Eighty-four percent of the population lives in rural areas. It is a "young country," as 45 percent of the population is under fifteen years of age. (1) It also is a very poor country. In early 2016 the World Bank gave Malawi its lowest global country ranking. (2) Despite these challenges, Malawi has made considerable improvements in rates of maternal and infant mortality over recent decades. The neonatal mortality rate per 100,000 live births was 21.8 in 2015, compared to 31.7 in 2002, and maternal mortality ratio per 100,000 live births fell from 1,100 in 1990 to 510 in 2013. (3)

The Ministry of Health is responsible for health care delivery in Malawi. Approximately 60 percent of health services are provided through government facilities, and the Christian Health Association of Malawi (CHAM) provides an additional 37 percent of Malawi's health care services. It also trains up to 80 percent of Malawi's health care providers. (4) Most health care is delivered at the primary care level in local health centers or dispensaries, with referrals made to district general hospitals or tertiary facilities. There are essentially no private-sector health services in the country.

This chapter describes an innovative cervical cancer screening program in a rural, poor area of Malawi. In particular, we discuss the feasibility of using thermo-coagulation to treat cervical lesions as an alternative to cryotherapy.

Case Study

The Nkhoma Cervical Cancer Screening Programme (Nkhoma CCSP), established in rural Central Malawi, represents an innovative way to address the high burden of cervical cancer in a poor, rural community. A program of cervical screening by visual inspection with acetic acid (VIA) and treatment of early lesions using thermo-coagulation was introduced in Nkhoma Hospital and surrounding health centers. One such health center is Chimbalanga, a small health facility lacking electricity, among other things that are taken for granted in the developed world. Chimbalanga is not easy to get to. With a team of Nkhoma VIA providers, we made the journey in a 4x4 Jeep across rough tracks that barely passed for a road. We took a portable generator, sterile specula, and all the other consumables needed to run a cervical cancer screening program in a rural setting. A weeklong screening campaign was organized for September/October 2015, the date being determined by the weather (before the rainy season) and the availability of local staff to help oversee the program.

We first conducted an educational campaign to spread the word about the program so as to encourage the local women to come get screened. On the first day, 53 women turned up, and the number increased each day, reaching a total of more than 400 women by the end of the week. Some women had to be turned away due to lack of sterile specula, as well as time! However, Nkhoma staff promised to return to Chimbalanga by the end of the month, and they did indeed return to screen an additional 198 women. Table 5.1 shows the results of the weeklong screening campaign.

We were very pleased by the response to the program. What made this campaign so successful, in our opinion, were positive word-of-mouth advocacy among the local women and the support of the program by the local village chief. For example, on the first day, one of the women who tested positive declined treatment, saying that she would have to first get her husband's permission to receive it. The clinic staff encouraged her to come back with her husband the following day for thermo-coagulation treatment. As it happens, her husband was the village chief, so perhaps obtaining his permission was necessary. However, no sooner had the woman left the clinic than she met her sister-in-law, the village chief's sister. Her sister-in-law immediately said that she should go right back and get the treatment, and she offered to talk to her brother to make sure that her sister-in-law received the necessary care. The village chief's wife did indeed return for treatment

Table 5.1. Number Screened and Treated in 2015

Day	Attending	First-ever screen	Given treatment on same day	Treatments postponed	Suspicious/ frank cancers
September 28	53	53	4	0	2
September 29	67	67	3	0	0
September 30	93	93	0	0	0
October 10	98	96	19	1	0
October 11	107	107	4	3	1

that day, along with her husband, who wanted to thank the clinic team for the good work they were doing. Thereafter this husband and wife team acted as advocates for screening and women's empowerment to make their own decisions. They have since spoken to various local groups about the importance of screening for cervical cancer.

The Burden of Cervical Cancer Screening in Low- and Middle-Income Countries and in Malawi

Cervical cancer is the most common cancer and the leading cause of cancer deaths among women in low- and middle-income countries (LMICs), and Malawi is no exception. (5) In the WHO African region in 2008, 75,000 new cases were recorded and more than 50,000 deaths. (6) This is probably an underestimate given the poor state of disease registries in most African countries. Despite the high burden of the disease, most LMIC countries do not provide cervical cancer prevention services. (7)

Malawi is a prime example of an LMIC trying to cope with a high incidence of cervical cancer. Malawi has one of the world's highest rates of cervical cancer; it is the most common female cancer in women fifteen to forty-four years old in Malawi, with an age-standardized rate of 75.9 per 100,000 population. (8) The cumulative risk of getting cervical cancer at seventy-five years of age in Malawi is 7.5 percent, compared to 1.4 percent globally. (9) An estimated 3,684 new cervical cancer cases were diagnosed in 2012, but this is also probably an underestimate. A national population-based cancer registry study of new cancer cases in Malawi from 2007 to 2010 found that cervical cancer accounted for 45.5 percent of all cancer incidence. (10) The high prevalence of cervical cancer is reflected in the caseload in pathology and palliative care services. (11,12)

There are serious challenges and barriers to organizing a cervical cancer screening program in LMICs. Chidyaonga-Maseko et al. (7) reviewed literature published since 2001 and described barriers to cervical screening in LMICs. They applied constant comparative analysis to identify thematic categories. Barriers identified included lack of or inadequate knowledge about cervical cancer, lack of familiarity with the concept of preventative health care, and geographic and economic inaccessibility to the screening services. Fear of a cervical cancer diagnosis and diffidence relating to the intimate nature of the screening procedure were also cited as barriers to screening. Stigma relating to women's reproductive health issues and taboos relating to cancer disclosure are important community-related factors that must be considered when designing a cervical cancer screening program. Limited or nonexistent access to and availability of services is a common barrier in almost all LMICs. The paucity of sufficient facilities providing screening services as well as trained personnel can be a huge barrier to care. Often educational programs and supportive programs are nonexistent, which can impede women from participating in a screening program even if it is available.

Maseko and colleagues (13) researched the challenges to delivering a cervical cancer prevention program in Malawi. They carried out a mixed-methods study to document health system gaps and identify challenges to the provision of cervical screening across the country. Responses to semi-structured questionnaires from district cervical cancer coordinators and service providers identified a number of health system concerns, primarily relating to workforce capacity and skill sets and the availability of essential medical products and treatment technologies. The authors reported a lack of an adequate, well-trained, evenly distributed, and well-supervised workforce, as well as a lack of basic provisions and medical consumables for screening and treatment in the local health facilities. They also noted the disparity in cervical screening provision between urban and rural areas in Malawi.

Another qualitative study of service providers cited a gross shortage of trained staff, lack of equipment and supplies, lack of supportive supervision, and use of male service providers. In addition, the lack of awareness of cervical cancer in the community, large distances to health facilities, and misconceptions about cervical cancer were noted. (14)

A number of recent studies have examined the understanding and attitudes of Malawian women regarding cervical cancer and screening. Maseko and colleagues (15) carried out a client satisfaction survey among 120 women recruited from sixteen screening centers across Malawi. They found overall high satisfaction with the service, but acknowledged that in the cultural context of low health care provision, women may have had low or no expectations to assess against.

Qualitative studies can often provide more in-depth perspectives. Fort and colleagues (16) studied rural women and identified barriers to seeking care, including lack of faith in the medical system, poor knowledge of cervical cancer, and poor insight regarding the benefits of screening. Cultural factors such as shame about being perceived as "sick" or being seen to be seeking medical care were also cited as common barriers. Other factors influencing screening attendance included a fatalistic view of cervical cancer, time pressures, childcare responsibilities, and fear of hidden costs of treatment. That being said, Ports and colleagues found a desire among women for health information, particularly from trusted medical sources, as well as an interest in community health advocacy and endorsement from local community leaders. (17)

Recognizing the growing incidence of cervical cancer in Malawi, in 2008 Mlombe and colleagues called for a national cancer strategy for Malawi. (18) They highlighted the lack of human papillomavirus (HPV) vaccination in the country and the need for a national cancer screening strategy. The Malawian Ministry of Health Strategic Plan 2011–2016 recommended that cervical screening use VIA and treatment of early lesions with cryotherapy as part of the national policy. This recommendation is in line with the World Health Organization's *Comprehensive Cervical Cancer Control: A Guide to Essential Practice.* (19,20) The Malawi plan, however, did not include recommendations about HPV vaccination.

A 2016 Ministry of Health policy briefing emphasized that a "screen and treat" approach using VIA is a cost-effective way to screen in low-resource settings such as Malawi. (21) Screen and treat bases the treatment decision on a screening test, with treatment provided immediately or at least soon after a positive screening test. This approach is particularly valuable in settings where women may not be able to return for treatment on another day. (22,23) Other recommendations from the briefing included ensuring that services are available at primary health care facilities; increasing the training, support, and supervision of more providers; increasing community awareness; and introduction of the HPV vaccine. (21) A new Malawi Strategic Plan for Cervical Cancer Prevention and Control 2016–2020 is under development and is expected to recommend widespread implementation of HPV vaccination, dependent on sufficient funding, as well as strengthening of cervical screening provision nationally. A complicating factor that must be considered is the high rate of HIV infection among Malawian women.

HIV and Cervical Cancer in Malawi

Like in much of sub-Saharan Africa, the high incidence of cervical cancer in Malawi is closely related to the high incidence of HIV infection. The prevalence of HPV infection and associated disease is also very high in HIV-infected individuals, even after antiretroviral therapy (ART) is started. It is estimated that one in twenty Malawi adults is on ART. (24) A systematic review of the literature shows that the average age at diagnosis of cervical cancer in HIV-positive women is ten years lower than among seronegative women. (25) HIV incidence in Malawi is estimated to be 10 to 12 percent in adults fifteen to forty-nine years old. The number of women age fifteen and older living with HIV is estimated to be 560,000. (26) HIV infection rates vary across the country and are higher in urban areas than in rural ones.

Regarding the relationship between HIV and cervical cancer, a recent review of pathology specimens in a Malawian hospital found that the likelihood of CIN2+ staged disease was over six times greater for HIV positive women. (27) We and others have shown high rates of high-risk HPV subtypes in HIV positive women in Malawi (28,29) and higher rates of VIA positivity in HIV positive women. (29,30) The integration of HIV/ART services and reproductive health services, including cervical screening, has been shown to be acceptable and has led to increased uptake of services. (31)

Malawi is currently implementing the 2015–2020 National HIV and AIDS Strategic Plan, (32) which aims to reduce HIV infections in line with the UNAIDS 90–90–90 targets (90% of people living with HIV will know their status, 90% of people diagnosed will be on ART, and 90% of people on ART will be virally suppressed). Chinula and colleagues argue that sustained investment in HIV-associated malignancies has the potential to improve care for both HIV positive and HIV negative patients, and certainly this is true with respect to cervical cancer. Strengthening ART services and linking them with robust cervical screening provision where HIV counseling and testing are also available should be strongly encouraged. (33)

HPV Vaccination and Cervical Cancer in Malawi

Cervical screening is only one component of a comprehensive cervical cancer prevention program. Immunization with one of the HPV vaccines should also be seriously considered. In Malawi, an HPV vaccination demonstration pilot was introduced in Rumphi and Zomba districts in 2013–2014 using a school-based approach targeting standard 4 girls nine to thirteen years old. The project was implemented with financial support from the Global Alliance for Vaccines and Immunization (GAVI) for procurement of HPV vaccines and supplies and in-kind support from the Malawian Ministry of Health. The project achieved vaccination coverage of almost 90 percent in both districts. This is a very impressive and encouraging figure. Although there are plans for further pilot work and a national scale-up of HPV vaccination, this is dependent on funding.

Challenges to Implementing Cervical Cancer Screening in Malawi

There are many challenges to implementing cervical screening in Malawi. A retrospective cohort study of cervical screening uptake from 2011 to 2015 written by key national screening stakeholders provides an informative overview of how the service has developed. It also provides valuable baseline data against which future interventions and initiatives can be measured, an important component of any program evaluation. (34) Findings show that by the end of 2015 the number of VIA sites increased to 130 — up from 75 in 2011 — of which 32 are established cryotherapy sites. However, only 22 of these cryotherapy sites were functional due to machine faults or lack of gas. In 2015 more than 44,000 Malawian women participated in a VIA screening program. Of these, 4.6 percent were VIA positive, yet less than half of these women actually received cryotherapy treatment. (34) It was in this context of high rates of cervical cancer and of HIV infection that the Nkhoma Cervical Cancer Screening Programme (Nkhoma CCSP) was established in 2013.

Nkhoma Hospital CCSP Program

Setting the Scene

The Malawi cervical cancer screening program was funded for three years by the Scottish government in collaboration with the Nkhoma CCAP Hospital (MW01 2013–2016). Nkhoma has a service level agreement with the government of Malawi Ministry of Health to provide referral services for a rural population of approximately 400,000, which covers parts of Dedza and Lilongwe districts. Nkhoma providers worked with local staff to organize Ministry of Health–sponsored VIA training courses and provide placements in the hospital for experiential training in VIA.

Our program's objective was to develop a sustainable program of cervical screening using VIA and HPV testing in rural Malawi. The main aim of the program was to establish VIA screening clinics in Nkhoma CCAP Hospital catchment area that would be staffed by trained clinical officers and nurse/midwives. Training in VIA was provided by the Ministry of Health. Completion of the Malawian Ministry of Health VIA course was a prerequisite for all providers in the program.

Health Centers and Outreach

Some of the facilities were mission based (CHAM), while others were government-run basic health centers; some were relatively accessible by road, while others were a considerable distance away or located on tracks that were impassable during the rainy season. Five health centers had begun weekly clinics by the end of 2014; an additional three clinics were in operation by the end of 2015. Intensive weeklong "campaigns" were held in three centers. Support from Nkhoma providers continued for at least a month after the regular clinics started, together with a monthly treatment clinic to prevent women having to travel to the hospital. Same-day treatment was therefore lower than in the hospital but still reached 84 percent across all centers.

A "hub and spokes" model (see figure 5.1) enabled consolidation of skills within the hospital team. Those trained developed the skills and confidence to educate their peers in the health centers. There are now approximately thirty trained providers associated with Nkhoma CCSP. This model has great potential for a roll-out to wider areas of Malawi and beyond. In fact, screening sites are now spread across Malawi (including Queen Elizabeth Central Hospital, in Blantyre in Southern Malawi; Partners in Hope in

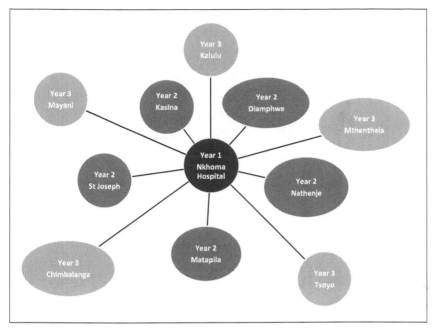

Figure 5.1. Hub and spokes model of service implementation in the Nkhoma CCSP

Madisi and Salima and Daeyang Luke Hospital in Central Malawi; and Karonga, Chitipa, Kasungu, Nkhota Kota, Dowa, and Mzuzu in the northern region).

Findings from Nkhoma CCSP

OUTCOMES BY AGE GROUP: In the first eighteen months (October 2013 to March 2015), 5,424 women presented for cervical cancer screening, of which almost 90 percent were first attenders. Of this number, 6.2 percent were known to be HIV positive. Among first attenders, 299 (6.3%) tested VIA positive. There were also 58 suspicious cancers identified that required a biopsy. Of the 58 women, 20 were diagnosed with advanced cancers. Pathways for intervention, including surgery and palliative care, were put in place. There is no chemo- or radiotherapy access in Malawi. (30)

Over the ensuing eighteen months Nkhoma CCSP introduced cervical screening to all the health centers within the catchment area. Data continue to be collected and pooled to provide program-level information. Figure 5.2 presents data on outcomes by age.

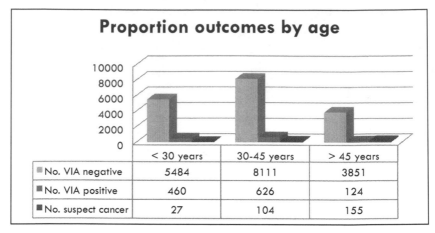

Proportion outcomes by age			
	< 30 years	30-45 years	> 45 years
▦ No. VIA negative	5484	8111	3851
▦ No. VIA positive	460	626	124
▪ No. suspect cancer	27	104	155

Figure 5.2. Nkhoma CCSP screening outcomes by age

From October 2013 to March 2016, more than 18,000 women were screened. Of these, over 8,000 (42.8%) were between the thirty and forty-five years old, the Malawi target age for cervical cancer screening. A number of older women with symptoms attended the screening service as a means of accessing health care. Both the Malawi Ministry of Health and Nkhoma CCSP have policies to screen any sexually active woman who requests it.

Although VIA negativity is high in all age cohorts, VIA positivity varied by age group: 7.7 percent among women under age thirty, 7.2 percent among those between thirty and forty-five, and only 3.0 percent among women over age forty-five. Not surprisingly, the incidence of suspected cancer is very low among the youngest women (0.45%), rising to 3.75 percent in over age forty-five.

OUTCOMES BY HIV STATUS: As mentioned previously, the risk of developing cervical cancer is high among women who are HIV positive. Figure 5.3 shows summary outcomes by HIV status in the Nkhoma CCSP between 2013 and 2016. As expected, findings showed that HIV positive women were at a greater risk of suspected cancer than non-HIV-infected women (2.8% versus 1.1%). Overall, among this screened population 5.6 percent of women were HIV positive, 51.7 percent were HIV negative, and HIV status was unknown in 42.7 percent. This is a lower rate of HIV infection than the national figure of 9.1 percent, and may reflect the rural location of our screened population. The proportion of women with unknown HIV status is expected to decrease in the coming years as Malawi implements the 90–90–90 plan.

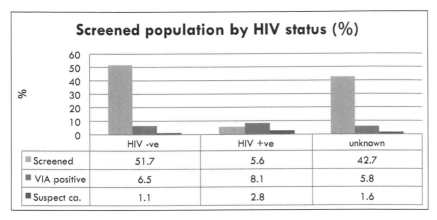

Figure 5.3 . Screening outcomes by HIV status

USE OF THERMO-COAGULATION: Since it is unethical to offer screening without ensuring follow-up treatment for those who test positive, we considered treatment options that would be feasible in a rural area. We needed to find alternatives to cryotherapy, a treatment recommended by the WHO for LMICs. We quickly found that cryotherapy was frequently not being done, partly due to lack of equipment and trained personnel and partly due to costs. It did not help that logistically it is very difficult to transport heavy cylinders to rural areas. Cold (thermo) coagulation, which is used in Scotland and elsewhere for low-grade lesions in young women, provided a suitable alternative for the Nkhoma program. (30,35) Thermo-coagulation is an ablative method for treatment of cervical intraepithelial neoplasia (CIN), and is suitable for use in LMICs. The equipment is small, portable, and durable. Abnormal cells are destroyed at 120°C in brief treatment applications using minimal electricity, and its use allows punch biopsies to be taken in the screening clinic.

Providers were trained in thermo-coagulation techniques. Each was required to have performed VIA screening on at least fifty women and to have performed ten thermo-coagulation treatments before his or her experiential training was considered complete. Where spaces in training sessions were available, the Nkhoma team has trained staff from other screening sites across Malawi in the use of thermo-coagulation, and several sites have now introduced thermo-coagulation into their treatment plans.

Given that thermo-coagulation was introduced as a replacement for cryotherapy, it was important to monitor outcomes among treated women.

All women receiving thermo-coagulation treatment are requested to return for a review visit between three and six months after treatment. In the first eighteen months of the program, 369 women received treatment with thermo-coagulation, 84 percent on the same day as the screening test. Of those treated, 234 women (63.4%) presented for a first follow-up visit between three and six months after treatment. On examination, the lesion was considered healed in 220 women (94%). A cure rate of 94 percent in this population is comparable to that found in the United Kingdom with the same treatment and is a comparable outcome to cryotherapy. Therefore we judge thermo-coagulation to be a noninferior treatment, suitable for use in this low-resource environment. (30,35)

Challenges Remain

Locally, Nkhoma CCSP has developed a model in which the Nkhoma Hospital works closely with the local health centers. Nonetheless, there still are a number of challenges that need to be addressed to maintain high-quality cervical cancer screening. Sustainability is a major issue. Ensuring a smooth flow of supplies and trained providers and retaining trained individuals to allow consistent, continuous delivery of services is a major challenge. Obtaining sufficient ongoing financing is a perennial challenge. However, we are pleased with how the program has grown.

Given the success of the Nkhoma CCSP project, we believe that the Malawi Ministry of Health could learn from the model to support wider implementation of cervical screening nationally with adequate financial support. For example, incorporating the screening program into existing reproductive health and HIV services would ensure that more women would be able to obtain access to health care, as well as streamline workforce and facility provision. Strategically, in Malawi as elsewhere, there needs to be awareness that the costs of cervical screening provision are matched by the costs of the cervical cancer burden, not just to the health system, but also to individual families and local economies. Indeed, consideration should be given to providing preventative health services such as screening for free in all government and CHAM health facilities.

We recognize that national implementation of such a program is a huge challenge for a poor country such as Malawi. Nationally, there remains a shortage of trained screening providers, especially in the rural health centers. Presently, trained personnel can be rotated or relocated to other parts of the country. Furthermore, there needs to be some sort of guaranteed supply of consumables such as cotton wool, vinegar, and gloves, which is a responsibility of local district health offices. Strategic investment in thermo-coagulators for district general hospitals across the country supporting local health centers (following the hub and spokes model outlined above) would also ensure that treatment would be available for VIA positive women.

In both rural and urban communities, there is still much work to be done to increase understanding of cervical cancer and the importance of cervical screening. The challenge is to translate that awareness into actual screening visits. Barriers include very practical work-home factors such as childcare and agricultural responsibilities, as well as fears and concerns based on low health literacy and charges. We recognize the need for ongoing awareness and educational messages that critically address myths and misconceptions held by many women in the rural communities. Nkhoma CCSP, for example, has worked with the hospital's drama group to develop culturally appropriate and acceptable drama skits and songs. Initiatives such as these should be expanded to spread the word.

Wider Public Health Context

While efforts are needed to address cervical screening capacity and the information needs of Malawian women, it is also important to acknowledge the wider public health context within which cervical screening is provided. Singh and colleagues (36) note the clear link in global inequalities between cervical cancer and disparities in human development as measured by the Human Development Index, social inequality including gender inequality, and national health care expenditure. While public health measures, including setting up cervical screening programs, public health education, and investment in vaccination, are critical, broader societal initiatives, including poverty reduction, expanding educational and economic opportunities for women, and a commitment to gender and social equality in the distribution of power, money, and resources, are also necessary.

Our Hopes for the Future

Given the high burden of cervical cancer in Malawi, we believe that priority should be given to improved provision of cervical cancer screening, as well as a national program of HPV vaccination targeting girls who are not yet sexually active. Immunization outreach, supported with good sexual health education, is critical. Yet, if an HPV vaccination policy was introduced immediately, there would still be a continued need for cervical screening.

Based on our experience, we strongly support the use of thermo-coagulation. We and others (Drs. R. Sankaranarayanan and J. Jeronimo, personal communications) are seeking to disseminate and develop the evidence base for this treatment modality because it is so suitable for low-resource facilities. The next generation of thermo-coagulators currently under development is smaller and either battery- or solar- powered, which would be most useful in a country like Malawi. Investment in thermo-coagulation as a treatment modality requires an initial capital outlay, but in our experience this is quickly balanced against the recurring costs of purchasing gas and cryoguns for cryotherapy.

The Nkhoma CCSP relies on VIA as the primary screening approach, but in keeping with developments in cervical screening worldwide, we recognize the potential of HPV testing and HPV immunization to transform cervical cancer screening in LMICs. We are exploring the use of HPV testing, as are other authors in this book. We strongly believe that HPV testing and HPV immunization hold great promise for significantly reducing the number of new cervical cancer cases among future generations of women, and Malawi is no exception.

References

1. World Health Organization. Malawi: WHO statistical profile [cited 2016 Dec 20]. Available from: http://www.who.int/gho/countries/mwi.pdf.

2. The World Bank. Data: Malawi [cited 2016 Dec 13]. Available from: http://data .worldbank.org/country/malawi.

3. World Health Organization. Countries: Malawi [cited 2016 Dec 13]. Available from: http://www.who.int/countries/mwi/en/.

4. Christian Health Association of Malawi [cited 2016 Dec 13]. Available from: http://www.cham.org.mw/.

5. Ferlay J, Soerjomataram I, Ervik M, et al. GLOBOCAN 2012, vol. 1.1: cancer incidence and mortality worldwide. IARC CancerBase No. 11. Lyon: International Agency for Research on Cancer; 2014 [cited 2016 Dec 13]. Available from: http:// globocan.iarc.fr.

6. Arbyn M, Castellsagué X, de Sanjosé S, et al. Worldwide burden of cervical cancer in 2008. Ann Oncol 2011;22(12):2675–86.

7. Chidyaonga-Maseko F, Chirwa ML, Muula AS. Underutilization of cervical

cancer prevention services in low and middle income countries: a review of contributing factors. Pan African Med J 2015;21:231. doi: 10.11604/pamj.2015.21.231.6350.

8. Forman D, Bray F, Brewster DH, et al., editors. Cancer incidence in five continents, Vol. X. IARC Scientific Publication No. 164. Lyon: International Agency for Research on Cancer; 2014.

9. Bruni L, Barrionuevo-Rosas L, Albero G, et al. ICO Information Centre on HPV and Cancer (HPV Information Centre): human papillomavirus and related diseases in Malawi. Summary Report. 2016 Oct 7 [cited 2016 Dec 13]. Available from: http://www.hpvcentre.net/statistics/reports/XWX.pdf.

10. Msyamboza KP, Dzamalala C, Mdokwe C, et al. Burden of cancer in Malawi; common types, incidence and trends: national population-based cancer registry. BMC Res Notes 2012;16(5):149. doi: 10.1186/1756-0500-5-149.

11. Gopal S, Krysiak R, Liomba NG, et al. Early experience after developing a pathology laboratory in Malawi, with emphasis on cancer diagnoses. PLoS One 2013; 8(8):e70361. doi: 10.1371/journal.pone.0070361.

12. Bates MJ, Mijoya A. A review of patients with advanced cervical cancer presenting to palliative care services at Queen Elizabeth Central Hospital in Blantyre, Malawi. Malawi Med J 2015;27(3):93–5.

13. Maseko FC, Chirwa ML, Muula AS. Health systems challenges in cervical cancer prevention program in Malawi. Glob Health Action 2015;8:26282. doi: 10.3402/gha.v8.26282.

14. Munthali AC, Ngwira BM, Taulo F. Exploring barriers to the delivery of cervical cancer screening and early treatment services in Malawi: some views from service providers. Patient Prefer Adherence 2015;9:501–8. doi: 10.2147/PPA.S69286.

15. Maseko FC, Chirwa ML, Muula AS. Client satisfaction with cervical cancer screening in Malawi. BMC Health Serv Res 2014;14:420. doi: 10.1186/1472-6963-14-420.

16. Fort VK, Makin MS, Siegler AJ, et al. Barriers to cervical cancer screening in Mulanje, Malawi: a qualitative study. Patient Prefer Adherence 2011;5:125–31.

17. Ports KA, Reddy DM, Rameshbabu A. Cervical cancer prevention in Malawi: a qualitative study of women's perspectives. J Health Commun 2015;20(1):97–104.

18. Mlombe Y, Othieno-Abinya N, Dzamalala C, Chisi J. The need for a national cancer policy in Malawi. Malawi Med J 2008;20(4):124–7.

19. The Malawi Health Sector Strategic Plan (HSSP) 2011–2016 [cited 2016 Dec 13]. Available from: http://www.nationalplanningcycles.org/sites/default/files/country _docs/Malawi/2_malawi_hssp_2011_-2016_final_document_1.pdf .

20. Comprehensive cervical cancer control: a guide to essential practice. 2nd ed. World Health Organization; 2014 [cited 2016 Dec 13]. Available from: http://apps.who .int/iris/bitstream/10665/144785/1/9789241548953_eng.pdf.

21. Phiri BC. Reducing cervical cancer prevalence in Malawi. Ministry of Health Policy Brief; 2016 Jul [cited 2016 Dec 13]. Available from: https://www.afidep.org /?wpfb_dl=190.

22. WHO guidelines for screening and treatment of precancerous lesions for

cervical cancer prevention. World Health Organization; 2014 [cited 2016 Dec 19]. Available from: http://apps.who.int/iris/bitstream/10665/94830/1/9789241548694_eng.pdf.

23. Denny L, Kuhn L, De Souza M, Pollack AE, Dupree W, Wright TC, Jr. Screen-and-treat approaches for cervical cancer prevention in low-resource settings. JAMA 2005;294(17):2173–81.

24. Government of Malawi. Malawi AIDS response progress report 2015. 2015 Apr [cited 2016 Dec 13]. Available from: http://www.unaids.org/sites/default/files/country/documents/MWI_narrative_report_2015.pdf.

25. Ntekim A, Campbell O, Rothenbacher D. Optimal management of cervical cancer in HIV-positive patients: a systematic review. Cancer Med 2015;4(9):1381–93.

26. UNAIDS. Malawi: HIV and AIDS estimates (2015) [cited 2016 Dec 13]. Available from: http://www.unaids.org/en/regionscountries/countries/malawi.

27. Kohler RE, Tang J, Gopal S, et al. High rates of cervical cancer among HIV-infected women at a referral hospital in Malawi. Int J STD AIDS 2015;27(9):753–60.

28. Cubie HA, Morton D, Kawonga E, et al. HPV prevalence in women attending cervical screening in rural Malawi using the cartridge-based Xpert HPV assay. J Clin Virol 2016 Dec 13. doi: 10.1016/j.jcv.2016.11.014.

29. Reddy D, Njala J, Stocker P, et al. High risk human papillomavirus in HIV-infected women undergoing cervical cancer screening in Lilongwe, Malawi: a pilot study. Int J STD AIDS 2015;26(6):379–87.

30. Campbell C, Kafwafwa S, Brown H, et al. Use of thermo-coagulation as an alternative treatment modality in a "screen-and-treat" programme of cervical screening in rural Malawi. Int J Cancer 2016;139(4):908–15.

31. Phiri S, Feldacker C, Chaweza T, et al. Integrating reproductive health services into HIV care: strategies for successful implementation in a low-resource HIV clinic in Lilongwe, Malawi. J Fam Plann Reprod Health Care 2016;42(1):17–23.

32. Malawi national HIV and AIDS strategic plan 2015–2020 [cited 2016 Dec 20]. Available from: http://hivstar.lshtm.ac.uk/files/2016/05/Malawi-National-HIV-AIDS-Strategic-Plan-2015-2020.pdf

33. Chinula L, Moses A, Gopal S. HIV-associated malignancies in sub-Saharan Africa: progress, challenges, and opportunities. Curr Opin HIV AIDS 2017;12(1): 89–95.

34. Msyamboza KP, Phiri T, Sichali W, et al. Cervical cancer screening uptake and challenges in Malawi from 2011 to 2015: retrospective cohort study. BMC Public Health 2016;16(1):806. doi: 10.1186/s12889-016-3530-y.

35. Dolman L, et al. Meta-analysis of the efficacy of thermo-coagulation as a treatment method for cervical intraepithelial neoplasia: a systematic review. BJOG 2014;121(8):929–42.

36. Singh GK, Azuine RE, Siahpush M. Global inequalities in cervical cancer incidence and mortality are linked to deprivation, low socioeconomic status, and human development. Int J MCH AIDS 2012;1(1):17–30

Chapter 6

Kaitlin McCurdy, Grace Tillyard, Joseph Bernard,
and Vincent DeGennaro Jr.

A National Cervical Cancer Screening
Program in Haiti

Introduction

Haiti has one of the highest rates of cervical cancer of any country in the world, with 94 cases per 100,000 population. Cervical cancer is the leading cause of cancer death in Haitian women, with an estimated 1,500 deaths annually. (1) This figure is probably an underestimate, given the difficulty in obtaining accurate morbidity and mortality counts, especially in the rural areas of the country. Considering the projected growth in the Haitian population, the number of women at risk for cervical cancer will certainly increase.

There are several small-scale screening programs throughout the country, but not enough to sufficiently reach the tens of thousands of women who should be screened. Innovating Health International (IHI), a nonprofit medical organization in Port Au Prince, Haiti, in collaboration with the Haitian Ministry of Health, set out to create an effective, national cervical cancer screening program in an effort to improve the early detection of cervical cancer and reduce the rate of invasive cervical cancer. This chapter discusses the key components of our national cervical cancer screening program, using our experience and the stories of our patients to describe our program and its potential impact. We also discuss the challenges to implementing screening programs in Haiti.

Case 1: Nadia—If Only She Had Gotten Screened

Nadia is a thirty-six-year-old woman who presented at our clinic one typical, hot Haitian morning. She waited her turn in line to see two doctors, one Haitian and one American. When it was her turn she sat down calmly and quietly and reported that she had started to experience some abdominal and lumbar back pain more than a year before. She also reported white vaginal discharge and scant vaginal bleeding for about the same length of time. She told the doctors that she had not been able to go to work for months because of her severe pain. A friend in her community told her that it could be an infection, so she took self-prescribed antibiotics instead of first consulting a physician. She had never had a Pap smear because she believed it was too expensive. She was a single mother of three children, and feeding them was her priority. She slowly handed the doctors a paper prescription that read "Stage IV Cervical Cancer, refer to IHI for palliative chemotherapy." She was not aware of what cervical cancer was until she was diagnosed with it, nor did she know that this type of cancer could be prevented by low-cost screening such as visual inspection with acetic acid (VIA). The doctors discussed the options with her and explained that they would set her up to begin treatment. They introduced her to the nurses who would be caring for her and the social worker who would pair her with a support buddy, a patient who had already gone through the journey she was about to embark upon. Radiation is not available in Haiti, and even if she were to seek treatment abroad, there was no one to care for her children. She also would be hard-pressed to pay for the treatment at all. Nadia's story is unfortunately not unique in Haiti. There are thousands of "Nadias" who cannot get the care that they need.

Background

Research clearly shows that oncogenic strains or high-risk strains of the human papillomavirus (HPV) cause cervical cancer. (2,3) In particular, HPV16 and HPV18 account for approximately 70 percent of this cancer. (4) Genital HPV types are categorized as low or high risk based on their oncogenic potential. Low-risk HPV types are typically associated with genital warts, whereas high-risk HPV types are associated with invasive cervical cancer. The most important causes of cervical cancer are persistent cervical infections caused by high-risk HPV (hrHPV) genotypes, in combination with a lack of access to preventive services.

Papanicolaou (Pap) testing remains the principle method to detect pre-cancerous lesions in women living in the developed world. However, its use in low- and middle-income countries (LMICs) is more problematic, if not impossible. Pap testing requires skilled practitioners, trained cytologists, a cytology lab, and the financial ability to pay for the test. Thus, to achieve high screening efficacy with Pap testing, a country must invest in adequate infrastructure (laboratories, diagnostic equipment, personnel, and so forth), which has been shown to be quite difficult in LMICs.

In many parts of the world, even some LMICs, the focus of efforts to stop cervical cancer is shifting toward prevention. This is not to say that screening will be eliminated; rather, with the development and implementation of prophylactic vaccines for primary prevention, young pre-sexually active girls can be immunized, thus substantially reducing their risk of developing cervical cancer later in life. (5) Vaccination can effectively prevent more than 90 percent of HPV infections. (6) While universal HPV vaccination is an important goal, this strategy unfortunately fails to account for those already infected by the HPV virus. (7,8) Even if HPV vaccination is immediately instituted throughout Haiti, there will still be several generations of at-risk women; tens of thousands of Haitian women would likely develop invasive cervical cancer before the impact of HPV vaccination is observed. In addition, the cost of the vaccine is a huge barrier (estimated at US$13 per vaccine), putting vaccination out of reach for the Haitian and many other LMIC governments. (9)

The use of molecular hrHPV testing for secondary prevention is a potentially highly successful and cost-effective intervention that can be utilized for the detection of precancerous cervical lesions and early invasive cervical cancers. Recent studies have shown that hrHPV testing has tremendous potential for use in screening for cervical cancer and could soon be the gold standard of care in cervical cancer screening, even in LMICs. hrHPV testing is more sensitive and reliable for detecting many types of cervical cancer than Pap testing, resulting in earlier detection of high-grade lesions as well as a higher negative predictive value against developing cervical cancer following a negative result. (10,11) Some countries with adequate Pap capabilities are turning to hrHPV testing as the primary screening method of choice. (12,13) hrHPV testing could do much to reduce the burden of cervical cancer globally. (14)

Results are read by machines rather than humans and therefore do not require trained laboratory staff or cytopathologists for interpretation, as does traditional Pap testing. Importantly, hrHPV can be self-collected via vaginal swabs, thus allowing privacy in self-screenings and avoiding the

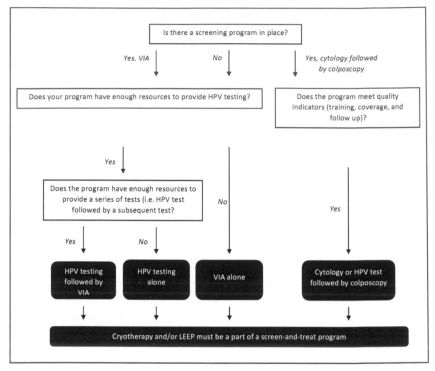

Figure 6.1. Decision-Making Flow Chart for Program Managers (extrapolated from the WHO recommendations)

discomfort of the pelvic examination. (15,16) In Haiti, Boggan et al. (17) found that self-administered vaginal hrHPV testing was concordant in detection with physician-administered cervical hrHPV testing. Their study was the first to show that self hrHPV testing is a feasible screening method for women in a low-resource Caribbean setting.

The World Health Organization (WHO) released new recommendations for cervical cancer screening and treatment in 2013 based on the utilization of two evidence-based techniques: hrHPV testing and VIA. (18) Cancer screening programs could use either hrHPV or VIA for initial screening and immediately treat anyone who screens positive ("screen and treat"). (See figure 6.1.) The WHO recommends hrHPV testing every three years for HIV-positive women and every five years for immune-competent women.

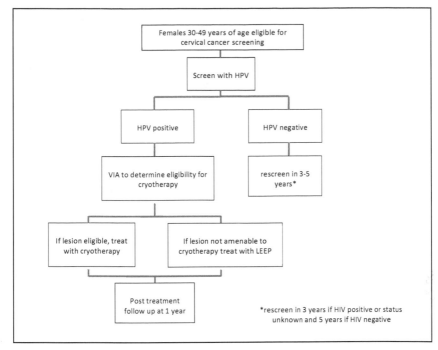

Figure 6.2. Recommended Cervical Cancer Screening in Haiti When HPV Testing Is Available

In Haiti, the Ministry of Health, Global Coalition Against Cervical Cancer, and IHI have adapted the WHO recommendations for cervical cancer screening. The Haitian program recommended that

- Women thirty to forty-nine years old should be screened with validated hrHPV tests at least once and no more than every three to five years, depending on HIV status (see figure 6.2).
- If hrHPV testing is not possible, women thirty to forty-nine years old should be screened with VIA at least once and no more than every three to five years, thereafter depending on HIV status (see figure 6.3).
- If feasible, women twenty-one to forty-nine years old should be screened by Pap test every three years.

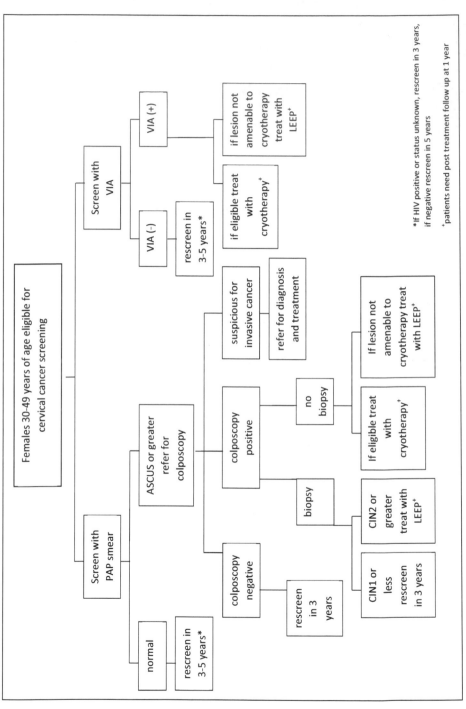

Figure 6.3. Recommended Cervical Cancer Screening in Haiti When HPV Testing Is Unavailable

The recommendations also include HPV vaccination for pre-sexually active individuals, but the Haitians acknowledge that a vaccination program is not possible with current resources.

Implementation of the Program

In 2015 IHI and the Haitian Ministry of Health received a grant to provide VIA and cryotherapy at eight of the largest hospitals, located in the geographic departments of Haiti. Obstetric nurses at each facility received training in VIA. When feasible at larger hospitals, colposcopy with loop electrosurgical excision procedure (LEEP) would be performed by an obstetrician trained in these techniques. To accomplish the overall goal, a four-phase plan was designed:

Phase 1: Train providers at eight departmental hospitals in VIA and cryotherapy in order to initiate a screen and treat strategy; Train obstetricians in colposcopy and LEEP techniques at the four largest departmental hospitals.

Phase 2: Introduce hrHPV screening in select departments.

Phase 3: Create national hrHPV testing coverage by expanding the screening program to reach all of Haiti, including outlying rural communities.

Phase 4: Start national HPV vaccination of all girls eleven to twenty-four years old.

In April 2016 the team launched Phase 1 goals in eight departmental hospitals. Supplies were obtained and allocated to each hospital. A dedicated training nurse was employed to provide a weeklong training session to four nurses and two doctors at each hospital. During this in-service training, 150 community patients were asked to volunteer to undergo screening in order to ensure that the obstetric staff obtained proficiency in performing VIA and cryotherapy. Training has been completed in five of eight locations, and active screening is ongoing in those five hospitals.

Haiti sans Cervical Cancer, a loose collection of nongovernmental organizations (NGOs), was formed with the mission of designing a "prevent and treat" cervical cancer network. Since each member organization already performs cervical cancer screening in different locations throughout the country, the goals of Haiti sans Cervical Cancer were to standardize screening protocols, simplify reporting to the Ministry of Health, improve patient navigation, procure supplies in bulk, and share best practices. Haiti sans Cervical Cancer partners has worked closely with IHI throughout the implementation of its cervical cancer screening program.

A standardized data collection sheet was designed and approved by Haiti sans Cervical Cancer. Each site utilized the same uniform data collection sheet to compile demographic and clinical information on all screened patients. Nurses performing VIA and cryotherapy enter data directly on the data collection sheet. The data are invaluable for evaluation and will give us insight into the actual incidence and prevalence of cervical cancer in our target population.

On average, our team visits each site every six weeks to monitor progress, address problems, exchange the CO_2 gas cylinders, inquire about supply usage, and review patient data. A designated training nurse at each site acts as a troubleshooter, checking on equipment problems, consulting on cases, and reinforcing support for the program. The training nurse visits the programs in the north during one week and those in the south during another week.

Colposcopy and LEEP are done only by OB-GYN or general surgeons; however, most of the major public hospitals only have part-time OB-GYN or general surgeons available. Training has lagged, as only two physicians have been trained to date. As a result few women have received colposcopy and/or LEEP at the public facilities. In many cases the lesions are amenable to cryotherapy. In other cases, the lesions are too advanced for LEEP or cryotherapy and require surgery. This situation is a huge problem and needs to be addressed. As the VIA/cryotherapy program expands and the number of women seen at each site increases, we expect that more cases of invasive cervical dysplasia or early cancers will be diagnosed, necessitating more physicians trained in colposcopy and/or LEEP. A sign of maturation in our program will be when 1 to 2 percent of all women screened do in fact undergo colposcopy/LEEP. We are a long way from reaching this goal, however.

Given the difficulty most of the poor, rural women have traveling to receive screening and treatment, we had to figure out how to offer basic treatment in each department. Those who require colposcopy and/or LEEP have to be referred to one of the four specialty centers. Women who require radical hysterectomy have to go to one of three hospitals, and those who require radiation have to be referred to the Dominican Republic or Cuba. The cost of obtaining these services, however, is considerable. Poor, rural women do not have the financial means, which is a huge barrier to receiving necessary treatment.

Phase II, slated to launch six months after Phase I, introduces hrHPV screening in two of the departments: Port-au-Prince and Cap Haitian. This phase includes working with private sector businesses to screen working-class women at their place of work.

Phase III focuses on scaling up HPV screening nationwide. Initially, we will utilize networks of clinics and hospitals that screen women using cervical or vaginal self-swabs, which are then taken by ground transportation to sites with HPV testing machines. The HPV samples are stable at room temperature without any preservative, which is important in a country such as Haiti. To achieve the goal of screening at least 80 percent of the female population, we will need to screen approximately 200,000 women per year. This will require coordinated efforts by multiple partners, including Haiti sans Cervical Cancer and the Ministry of Health.

Phase IV focuses on implementing a national hrHPV vaccination program for girls between eleven and twenty-four years old (approximately 1 million young women). No date has yet been set for this because the vaccine cold chain storage in Haiti is currently not sufficient. In addition, funding such a project is uncertain as of this writing.

Future Plans for Cervical Cancer Screening in Haiti

Our next steps will be to try to expand HPV testing nationwide, either by increasing the number of HPV testing machines in Haiti or simply by shipping samples from more clinics around the country to sites that already have the machines. We hope to expand our HPV screening program from two hospitals to four, but challenges must be addressed before we can implement any program expansion. Community-based outreach in churches and schools, for example, could be an effective way to educate and encourage women, especially in rural areas, to self-screen using vaginal swabs. A doctor and a nurse would not be required under such a scheme. In addition, urban women could self-screen at their workplace. Using vaginal self-swabs could be an effective way to expand the program. (See chapter 7, which details the Honduras program.)

In Haiti, HPV vaccination has been discussed at the ministry level since 2015. Given that many Haitians would not be able to afford the cost of the vaccine, there is a need for the government to subsidize the cost. The Global Alliance for Vaccines and Immunizations (GAVI) has helped subsidize the cost in many LMICs, but to be eligible for assistance from GAVI, Haiti must first meet benchmarks for pediatric vaccines to prove that cold-chain capacity exists to provide the vaccine. Haiti would be hard-pressed to meet such benchmarks at this time.

In addition to the cost of the vaccine, awareness is a barrier in Haiti. Fewer than one-quarter of Haitian women have heard of HPV, and only 10 percent have heard of the HPV vaccine. However, Gichane et al. (19) found that after an education program, more than 96 percent of Haitian mothers reported that if they were offered the vaccine for their daughters they would accept, and most Haitian mothers would be willing to pay $4.65 for the vaccination, an amount higher than the minimum wage for a day's work in the Haitian garment industry.

Case 2: Mireille and Joanne—Saved by Screening

Mireille is a fifty-two-year-old married woman with two children. She presented to the clinic, and the Haitian physician pointed out her address on the new patient form: "She came a long way. It took an entire day of travel." She reported that her symptoms started as pain during sexual intercourse, and she had heard through village elder women that this could be from her "female parts." So when she heard that free female exams were going on at the local departmental hospital, she went. Her VIA was positive, and she was referred to an OB-GYN. She had stage I cervical cancer and successfully underwent a radical hysterectomy. At follow-up appointments she told us how blessed she felt that her cancer was diagnosed at an early and treatable stage. She had known women who had not been so lucky and had passed away from cervical cancer. She wanted to give back to the cancer program, so we introduced her to our social worker. Mireille, now cancer free, is a leader in our community health worker group, called the Women's Health Promoters (WHP), which is dedicated to promoting cancer awareness to Haitian women and to encouraging women to get screened.

Joanne is thirty-four years old and was diagnosed with stage III breast cancer. She is now in remission and leading the charge as a member of the WHP for IHI's awareness program for breast and cervical cancer in Haiti. She first noticed a mass in her breast and bloody nipple discharge, which was present for eight months before she sought any sort of care. She had two separate biopsies at the main public hospital in Port-au-Prince in September and October 2015. She then came to the IHI Women's Cancer Program and had a mastectomy in March 2016, followed by chemotherapy through the summer of 2016. Since finishing chemotherapy, Joanne has been an active member of the support group of 130 patients and also serves as a Women's Health Promoter in her community. In only two months she has directed five awareness seminars in the community, at three churches, a school, and a health center, located in three different towns.

Joanne says, "I wanted to participate to improve awareness about cancer. I didn't know that blood coming from the nipple was a sign of cancer. If I had known that, I would have gone to see the doctor sooner. I want women to learn from me because I know that I wouldn't have had such an advanced cancer if I had been educated like these women who benefit from our awareness program." Now she encourages screening, and refers any friends or women in the community to the nearest doctor for evaluation. She is a leader in her community, and for all that she does, she still feels that more needs to be done. "IHI will motivate women with our program. But it's not enough; one-hour sessions are too short. I often talk to one woman on the street for an hour about cancer and their symptoms."

Joanne understands how difficult it is to convince women to get screened for something when they have no symptoms. Many women in Haiti don't see a doctor until they have symptoms, which is often too late. Furthermore, many don't know that cancer is a disease; many believe the word cancer is only used to describe a "negative person" in the community. "IHI have to educate them on what cancer is first, and then convince them of the value of screening."

Awareness and Engagement

To increase acceptance and utilization of cervical cancer screening and to encourage self-breast exam, IHI designed a communications toolkit and engaged breast cancer patients and survivors as women's health promoters in their communities. Joanne is one of the women's health promoters and regularly encourages women with signs of cancer, such as lumps in the breast and vaginal bleeding, to be screened. The efforts of the WHP have led to a doubling of the number of new cases of breast cancer at the Women's Cancer Treatment Center operated by IHI in Port-au-Prince, Haiti.

Widespread education, awareness, and engagement are key components of screening and early detection programs targeting cervical and breast cancer. Low levels of education and lack of engagement in many low-income countries lead to poor adherence rates, refusal to undergo lifesaving treatment, and poor outcomes. There is increasing evidence that health communication and education can foster greater community engagement and improve health, particularly through community-based initiatives that conduct outreach and connect people in poor or rural communities with screening and treatment facilities. (20–23) Evidence-based approaches and community involvement are essential to the success of any awareness- and engagement-raising public health initiatives. It is equally essential that education programs go beyond addressing conventional understanding of barriers to care. They must also address social and cultural concerns, or the utilization of services will continue to be low despite availability and good access.

Challenges Remain

Haiti can learn from other LMICs. Many low-income countries are attempting both high-tech and low-tech solutions to increasing awareness. For example, the Uganda Women's Cancer Support Organization uses community support groups, led by local survivors of breast cancer, to increase awareness on a community level. Its newest project aims to address metastatic breast cancer through quality of life improvements. (24) The Institute for the Evaluation of Quality and Awareness in Health in Colombia has created a website in Spanish tailored to patients and caregivers on metastatic breast cancer that is applicable across Spanish-speaking countries in Latin America. (25) In Peru, the National Council for Science, Technology and Technological Innovation, in collaboration with Cayetano University School of Public Health, relies on women's health promoters to distribute self-administered vaginal swabs for HPV testing in the slum areas of Lima. Community-based collection points have been established, and the swabs are transported to a lab for analysis.

Despite the slowly expanding availability of screening in Haiti, there is a lack of awareness and outreach programs in the country, and women continue to present with advanced disease. Of the women diagnosed with cervical cancer through IHI's cancer treatment program, 75 percent have had stage III or IV cancer, and nearly all of them have presented after progressing beyond stage IIA, the stage at which they would still be eligible for radical hysterectomy instead of radiation. In our breast cancer program, 79 percent of women present in stage III and IV, and the mortality rate is high (24 percent in 2015). (26) These statistics show a need for increased engagement, collaboration, and trust among individuals, community leaders, health care providers, and the government. Many low-income countries have noted similar issues with lack of education and exposure, and cancer control will remain elusive if education and engagement are not prioritized.

In September 2015 IHI, in cooperation with the Haitian Support Group Against Cancer (GSCC) and five other local partners, implemented a women's cancer awareness and engagement campaign supported by the Union of International Cancer Control (UICC) and other donors. The program sought to address the issues of late presentation and lack of engagement by: increasing early cancer diagnosis; improving patient navigation in the health care system; encouraging patient input in the design and delivery of communication and awareness raising; and building local capacity by working with community-based organizations, local NGOs, and relevant government counterparts. The consortium accomplished these goals by creating the WHP, whose members have worked with us to create materials that reflect their experiences. These women act as ambassadors in their communities, linking their neighbors and friends to treatment centers. To aid the women in communicating with their communities, IHI created a toolkit designed to promote screening and early diagnosis of women's cancers.

IHI used community-based participatory research (CBPR) to implement a mixed-methods inquiry that included both closed and open-ended questions. A community advisory board (CAB), consisting of five civil society organizations, women's organizations, and representatives from the Ministry of Health, helped frame the questions deemed important based on focus group feedback. We focused on four important topics: demographics, knowledge and beliefs about the disease, relationship with health care infrastructure, and where people go to obtain information about health concerns. There were 414 participants from four of the ten geographic departments. Of these, 75 percent were women, and participants ranged in age from thirteen to sixty-five years.

Findings showed that for cervical cancer, both males and females had poor knowledge of the disease. Women stated more often than men that they know about risk factors; when asked to name some risk factors, responses included early sexual debut, many sexual partners, and vaginal infections. Only one woman mentioned HPV as a risk factor, and only three women specifically mentioned the man's role in transmitting the cancer. Other responses included rough sex and sexual positions as perceived causes of cervical cancer. The location of the cervix was identified correctly by only twenty-six respondents, while fifty-four knew it was part of the reproductive system. And 240 individuals did not know what the cervix is.

Only 22 percent reported knowing complications of cervical cancer. The most common complications noted from qualitative responses and focus groups were death, surgery to remove the uterus, and infertility. When questioned about diagnosing cervical cancer, only 12 percent reported knowing what a test for cervical cancer was, but 33 percent said they knew where to get a test for cervical cancer. However, women were less likely to seek out a test that they were not sure about, even if they knew where to get tested.

In general, males expressed resistance to cervical cancer screening. The impact of gender inequality and gender-based violence needs to be better understood in Haiti. Women who are victims of sexual and gender-based violence could be more vulnerable to developing cervical cancer. (27) To investigate further, IHI conducted a smaller, separate survey of fifty women who were being treated for breast cancer. Findings showed that 40 percent admitted to being victims of economic, psychological, sexual, and/or physical violence. This figure is significantly higher than the 28 percent of all women in the general population in Haiti that have been subjected to violence at some point in their lives after the age of fifteen. This finding needs to be more fully explored, especially since two weeks of sexual abstinence is required after undergoing cryotherapy or LEEP, which many partners refuse to grant to the woman. To what extent does this impact a woman's ability to receive potentially lifesaving treatment? Theoretically, some women would not be permitted to undergo a lifesaving procedure because their husbands or male partners refused to abstain from sex for two weeks.

The CAB and IHI used the survey results to design the communication and education toolkit for breast and cervical cancer with the trained women's health promoters. These women strongly suggested that we use the stories of those who have had breast cancer. The educational materials were designed to reflect the women's experiences and focused on intimate partner violence. IHI found narrative and empathy to be key motivators for other women to seek screening and treatment. The toolkit includes a manual for community health workers to learn about breast and cervical cancer, a patient education and orientation tool with visuals for breast and cervical cancer, a series of television spots featuring the members of the WHP as actresses, and a set of educational playing cards. These materials are not only "culturally relevant" but also reflect Haitian women's experiences with cancer.

IHI, with the guidance of the CAB, plans to continue to train local and international organizations working in Haiti. All the materials have been made open access and can be found on IHI website (www.innovatinghealth-international.org).

Joanne and thirty other breast cancer survivors who have been trained as women's health promoters in their communities constitute an essential bridge between health services in low-resource settings and the local community. The program has been successful in empowering these women to act as focal points in their community for other women who may have breast or gynecological problems. The program is entirely voluntary, and the women speak about their experiences as a means of educating their neighbors and friends about cancer. They are active in their churches and schools and utilize the media, including local radio. As stated previously, the WHP has helped IHI's clinics more than double the number of women diagnosed with breast cancer, which demonstrates the effectiveness of community-based interventions. Furthermore, the program was designed and implemented by a communication and service designer and a Haitian social worker, pointing to the importance of interdisciplinary and transnational thinking to solve public health problems in LMICS.

What Does the Future Hold for Cancer Screening in Haiti?

Cost and sustainability are constant problems in LMICs such as Haiti, where there are limited resources. Thinking creatively to survive financially is a necessity. In its cervical cancer screening program, IHI has left the model of implementation and cost recovery up to each individual hospital, but each asks for a small fee from the woman screened (less than $2) to purchase more supplies and pay the screening nurses' salaries. Each hospital program would need to screen 500 to 600 women per month to ensure sustainability at the end of the IHI grant period. Currently, no hospital is close to meeting this target, but we are hopeful that it will be reached.

The geography of Haiti is also a challenge. Mountainous terrain and poor road infrastructure complicate the transportation of supplies and the tanks of CO_2 for cryotherapy. One location in the Northwest department is a six-hour drive from the nearest gas distributor, most of which is over unpaved mountain roads. As a result, we decided to deliver two full tanks at a time while picking up the two empty tanks and to deliver tanks to all sites in the North during one trip and all the sites in the South during another trip. We had initially hoped to use a technology that didn't require gas cylinders (using electricity to freeze the probe instead of gas), but the equipment is still in the prototype phase and not available. Also, electricity can be unreliable in rural Haiti. When it becomes possible, we plan on using the equipment at the farthest sites to avoid having to deliver gas cylinders to such remote areas.

In addition, there is a paucity of trained gynecologic oncologists in Haiti, and the issue of provider availability won't be corrected anytime soon. According to the WHO, general OB-GYN physicians' training does not include performing radical hysterectomies, the treatment of choice in cases of Stage I or IIa cervical cancer. Staging of cervical cancer in Haiti is also a problem. Staging by CT scans, cystoscopy, and/or recto-sigmoidoscopy is next to impossible in Haiti outside of Port-au-Prince.

Another challenge we often witness is patients having difficulty navigating the medical system to find doctors who provide cancer care, both preventative and treatment. For example, the IHI clinic in Port-au-Prince provides patient consultation and chemotherapy under the supervision of two full-time internal medicine physicians. However, there is no on-site OB-GYN, and therefore any woman with suspected or confirmed cervical cancer must be referred to an alternative hospital with an OB-GYN physician on-site. Unfortunately the barriers to pursuing this referral are numerous; fewer than 40 percent of women we refer to the alternative hospital are ever evaluated by the physician. Reasons that women are lost to follow-up prior to evaluation by an OB-GYN include lack of funding (initial physician consultation costs 300 Haitian gourdes or US$5), difficulty in obtaining an appointment, transportation challenges, fear, and social repercussions/stigma.

We found that the greatest barrier to the treatment of advanced cervical cancer in Haiti is the absence of radiation therapy. As stated previously, patients must be referred to the Dominican Republic or Cuba to receive such treatment. However, the total cost, including radiation, travel, and lodging, is usually over US$2,000, far out of reach of all but the wealthy. Obtaining Haitian passports is complex for those without birth certificates or voting cards, and Dominican visas are limited in number. Over the past three years, of the roughly one hundred women we have treated for cervical cancer who needed radiation therapy, only four have successfully received treatment in a neighboring country. The treatment requires that the individual spend four to six weeks out of the country, more often than not without family members to help care for them throughout the arduous process.

Screening for breast cancer relies on either breast self-exam or breast exam by a nurse or physician. However, follow-up treatment, such as surgery, radiation, and chemotherapy, is very limited and very costly.

Our screening program also encountered a number of other barriers, both natural and man-made. The October 2015 Haitian elections were invalidated due to accusations of fraud, and a transitional government was put in place months later (in February 2016). Higher-level Ministry of Health employees, all political appointees, turned over as a result of the change in government, interrupting continuity of leadership and logistics and leaving the program without a champion within the central ministry. We have since operated under regional and hospital-based implementation arrangements. In addition, a national physician strike lasted from May to September 2016, which closed all major public hospitals across the entire country, making it impossible to implement or carry out existing programs anywhere in Haiti.

Also in 2016, Hurricane Matthew, a category 5 Atlantic hurricane, slammed into the southern peninsula of Haiti, killing well over a thousand people and leaving a large majority of survivors without shelter, food, or clean water. IHI temporarily suspended all noncritical activities to assist in medical disaster relief in the affected regions. Due to Hurricane Matthew, there was an indefinite delay in training and screening in three of the main public hospitals, which were rendered temporarily nonfunctional. We are slowly resuming the program, although post-hurricane-related problems persist.

Concluding Thoughts

Cervical cancer is the leading cause of cancer and cancer-related death in Haiti. But breast cancer, too, is prevalent in Haiti. IHI believes that there is a great opportunity to support innovative programs in cancer screening in Haiti despite the challenges. Along with the Ministry of Health and Haiti sans Cervical Cancer, IHI has begun implementing a nationwide initiation of screen and treat cervical exams using VIA and cryotherapy followed by colposcopy and/or LEEP, with some degree of success. Barriers to treatment for breast cancer have proven to be more difficult to overcome. Challenges certainly remain. However, our future plans include broadening hrHPV testing and initiating nationwide HPV vaccinations. Though we have encountered many challenges in this unique, poor country, we remain optimistic and are encouraged by the patients whose lives we have impacted and the stories they live to share.

References

1. Ferlay J, Soerjomataram I, Ervik M., et al. GLOBOCAN 2012 v1.0, cancer incidence and mortality worldwide: AIRC CancerBase No. 11. Lyon, France: International Agency for Research on Cancer; 2013 [cited 2016 Dec 20]. Available from: http://www.globocan.iarc.fr.

2. World Health Organization. Cancer fact sheet [cited 2016 Dec 20]. Available from: www.who.int/mediacentre/factsheets/fs297/en/.

3. Torre LA, Siegel RL, Ward EM, and Jemal A. Global cancer incidence and mortality rates and trends—an update. Cancer Epidemiol Biomarkers Prev 2016;25:16–27.

4. GHESKIO Centers. Cervical cancer in Haiti [cited 2016 Dec 20]. Available from: Gheskio.org/wp/?page_id=336.

5. Schiffman M, Castle PE, Jeronimo J, et al. Human papillomavirus and cervical cancer. Lancet 2007;370(9590):890–907.

6. Forman D, de Martel C, Lacey CJ, et al. Global burden of human papillomavirus and related diseases. Vaccine 2012;30(Suppl 5):F12–23. doi: 10.1016/j.

7. de Sanjose S, Quint WG, Alemany L, et al. Human papillomavirus genotype attribution in invasive cervical cancer: a retrospective cross-sectional worldwide study. Lancet Oncol 2010;11(11):1048–56.

8. Petrosky E, Bocchini JA, Hariri S, et al. Use of 9-valent human papillomavirus (HPV) vaccine: updated HPV vaccination recommendations of the Advisory Committee on Immunization Practices. Morb Mortal Wkly Rep 2015;Mar 27;64(11):300–4.

9. Cutts FT, Francesch S, Goldie, S et al. Human papillomavirus and HPV vaccine: a review. Bull of WHO [cited 2016 Dec 20]. Available from: www.who.int/bulletin/volumes85/9/06-038414/en/.

10. Garland SM, Hernandez-Avila M, Wheeler CM, et al. Quadrivalent vaccine against human papillomavirus to prevent anogenital diseases. N Eng J Med 2007; 356(19):1928–43.

11. Hildesheim A, Herrero R, Wacholder S, et al. Effect of human papillomavirus 16/18 L1 viruslike particle vaccine among young women with preexisting infection: a randomized trial. JAMA 2007;298(7):743–53.

12. Wigle J, Coast E, Watson-Jones D. Human papillomavirus (HPV) vaccine

implementation in low and middle-income countries (LMICs): health system experiences and prospects. Vaccine 2013;31(37):3811–7.

13. Ronco G, Dillner J, Elfstrom KM, et al. Efficacy of HPV-based screening for prevention of invasive cervical cancer: follow-up of four European randomised controlled trials. Lancet 2013;(13)62218–7 [cited 2017 Sep 1]. Available from: http://dx.doi.org/10.1016/S0140-6736(13)62218-7.

14. Sankaranarayanan R, Nene BM, Shastri SS, et al. HPV screening for cervical cancer in rural India. N Eng J Med 2009;360(14):1385–94.

15. Saslow D, Solomon D, Lawson HW, et al. American Cancer Society, American Society for Colposcopy and Cervical Pathology, and American Society for Clinical Pathology screening guidelines for the prevention and early detection of cervical cancer. CA Cancer J Clin 2012;62(3):147–72.

16. The Dutch National Institute for Public Health and the Environment. Cervical cancer screening in the Netherlands. 2014 [cited 2017 Sep 1]. Available from: http://www.rivm.nl/en/Documents_and_publications/Common_and_Present/News messages/2014/Cervical_cancer_screening_in_the_Netherlands.

17. Schiffman M, Castle PE. The promise of global cervical-cancer prevention. N Eng J Med 2005;353(20):2101–4.

18. Arbyn M, Verdoodt F, Snijders PJ, et al. Accuracy of human papillomavirus testing on self-collected versus clinician-collected samples: a meta-analysis. Lancet Oncol 2014;15(2):172–83.

19. Arbyn M, Castle PE. Offering self-sampling kits for HPV testing to reach women who do not attend in the regular cervical cancer screening program. Cancer Epidemiol Biomarkers Prev 2015;24(5):769–72.

20. Boggan J, Walmer D, Henderson G, et al. Vaginal self-sampling for HPV infection as a primary cervical cancer screening tool in a Haitian population. Sex Trans Dis 2015;42(11):655–9.

21. World Health Organization. Guidelines for screening and treatment of precancerous lesions for cervical cancer prevention [cited 2016 Dec 20]. Available from: www.who.int/reproductivehealth.

22. Gichane MW, Calowa MW, McCarthy SH, et al. Human papillomavirus awareness in Haiti: preparing for a national HPV vaccination program. J Pediatr Adolesc Gynecol 2017;30(1):96–101.

23. O'Neil DS, Lam WC, Nyirangirimana P, et al. Evaluation of care access and hypertension control in a community health worker driven non-communicable disease programme in rural Uganda: the chronic disease in the community project. Health Policy Plan 2016;Mar 8(pii): czw006.

24. UWOCASO. Uganda women's cancer support organization [cited 2016 Dec 20]. Available from: Uwocaso.org.ug.

25. UNESDOC. National Accreditation System in Colombia. 2003 [cited 2016 Dec 20]. Available from: http://unesdoc.unesco.org/images/0013/001310/131066e.pdf.

26. Gomez A, DeGennaro V, George SHL, et al. Presentation, treatment and

outcomes of Haitian women with breast cancer in Miami and Haiti: Disparities in breast cancer—a retrospective cohort study. J Global Oncol 2016 Nov 2.

27. United Nations Population Fund. Addressing violence against women and girls in sexual and reproductive health services: a review of knowledge assets [cited 2016 Dec 20]. Available from: www.unfpa.org/sites/default/files/pub-pdf/addressing _violence.pdf.

Chapter 7

Linda S. Kennedy and Gregory J. Tsongalis

Case Study

Introducing PCR Testing for
High-Risk HPV in Honduras

H onduras, located in Central America, has a population of 8 million
people, approximately half of whom reside in rural areas, where the
majority of households meet the criteria for living in extreme poverty (defined as living on less than US$2.50 per day). (1) Economi-
cally, Honduras is the second poorest country in the Western Hemisphere;
Haiti is the poorest. (2) There is a long-standing tradition in Honduras of
free "brigade-style" medical care staffed by international medical teams.
Medical brigades work with licensed medical professionals and community
health workers to provide expanded health services in rural communities
with limited access to health care. For example, the government's national
vaccine program achieves nearly 90 percent compliance annually. (3)

The Burden of Cervical Cancer: Focus on Honduras

Many cervical cancer screening programs have been developed around the
globe in an effort to reduce the morbidity and mortality from this disease.
Though cervical cancer is both preventable and curable, the mortality rate
is high among women living in low- and middle-income countries (LMICs),
primarily due to the advanced stages the disease has reached at presentation. Sankaranarayanan's (4) review of cancer screening in LMICs dis-
tinguishes between "organized" and "opportunistic" screening programs,
with organized screening characterized by targeted populations, planned

follow-up, and research investigations combined with clinical follow-up. Opportunistic screening includes programs that are unorganized at the local level or spontaneously add screening tests when people seek medical care for other reasons. (4) Factors such as geography, accessibility, availability of personnel, logistics, and other site-specific, resource-limited, or culturally specific factors need to be considered when designing the nature and scope of a screening program.

Honduras has a population of 2.78 million women age fifteen and older who are at risk of developing cervical cancer. Although screening by Pap smear is mandated by the Honduran national cancer program for targeted segments of the population, only 10 percent of women of screening age (defined by Honduras as eighteen to seventy years old) are tested each year. Honduras, like many LMICs, has no national cancer or screening registry; it is not possible to know to what extent the 10 percent who are screened each year are the same women. (5) Furthermore, there is a serious lack of capacity to evaluate Pap smears due to the paucity of pathologists and cytologists in the country. Typically, Honduran women wait at least six months to receive results of their Pap screening (6), in contrast to the United States, where the turnaround time is three to four days. Yet previous community-based education about cervical cancer screening in Honduras showed it to be effective and inexpensive. (7) Of note, in 2016 a human papillomavirus (HPV) vaccine pilot program for girls nine to eleven years old was initiated, which prospectively should help curb the incidence of this cancer in Honduran women.

In the past decade, the quickly changing landscape of cervical cancer screening in LMICs has included traditional Pap smear testing, with its reliance on well-trained yet generally scarce pathologists, as well as visual inspection with ascetic acid (VIA), which can be performed by trained nonphysician providers. More recently, cervical cancer screening has advanced to molecular testing by PCR (polymerase chain reaction) for high-risk human papillomavirus (hrHPV) detection, which reduces the workload for pathology by alleviating the need for subsequent Pap screening of women who are found to be hrHPV negative. Currently, Honduran public health officials have had to rely on estimated rates of infection by hrHPV when making difficult decisions about use of scarce resources for cervical cancer screening or prevention programs. (8) An evidence-based, feasible, acceptable, and cost-effective program to prevent cervical cancer that relies on some combination of vaccination and screening is essential to reduce the cancer burden in Honduras

This case study describes the Dartmouth Norris Cotton Cancer Center's (NCCC) development of an organized cervical cancer screening research program in Honduras that focuses on testing women for hrHPV using the new molecular technology. As conceived, the NCCC protocol focused on utilizing new assays to determine all hrHPV types present in a patient sample. This is key information for epidemiologists tracking disease geographically and for policy makers considering investment in and deployment of vaccines on a population level. The project sought to address the following:

1. Feasibility of brigade-style screening adapted to cervical cancer screening.
2. Feasibility of high-tech PCR screening systems performing to standards in challenging environmental conditions.
3. Most important, the extent to which women would choose to participate in cervical cancer screening if it were made available.

To adequately address these questions and operationalize the research protocol, NCCC began the process of developing collaborative relationships for a research infrastructure in Honduras. Our team from NCCC decided on a strategy to locate the screening programs in a crowded urban maquila (factory) and a rural, poor village. Central to the protocol was a rapid, accurate, inexpensive PCR assay to simultaneously test for all fourteen known types of hrHPV. For the rural program, we transported the PCR instrumentation in an ordinary pick-up truck over difficult terrain and gave intensive short-term training to Honduran pathologists who would be hands-on technicians. The protocol met the criteria of quick turnaround time for results and added the benefit of rapid throughput due to its capacity to concurrently process ninety-six specimens (ninety-four patient samples and two controls). Because HPV-based screening alone has a low positive predictive value for cervical cancer, (9) the protocol screened for hrHPV and used reflexive Pap smear testing to assess for pre- or invasive cervical cancer. When identified early, pre- or invasive cervical cancer can often be treated successfully in a doctor's office or clinic setting. All program material was translated into Spanish. We followed the standards for screening in LMICs. (10) Institutional review board (IRB) approval was granted by Dartmouth College and the Universidad de Catolica in Honduras.

Building a Partnership

The decision to focus NCCC's research efforts primarily in one country was a practical one. It is a significant challenge to build an infrastructure of personal connections for collaborative research, including such critical elements as IRB approval, shipping biological specimens, quality control, and developing welcoming sites for clinical trials with local partners. Since its inception in 2012, NCCC's work in Honduras has relied on a comprehensive approach of team science and the ethic of sharing opportunities for investigation, data, and equipment. By developing authentic partnerships with Hondurans ranging from oncologists and medical faculty, to village leaders and the government's social security medical program, the underpinnings of the infrastructure began to form.

The goal was to foster collaborative team science. For example, targets for study were discussed with both strategic and opportunistic options in mind. From the outset, using a model of community-led action research, NCCC cultivated an increasingly strong partnership among colleagues from NCCC and Honduras, each contributing significantly to the selection of targets and formulation of research questions. Each person in the evolving research group brought expert knowledge from a different perspective; the end result was that the synthesis of ideas was far more nuanced than either institution could have achieved on its own.

At a seminal meeting held in 2012, NCCC investigators and Honduran oncologists discussed for the first time the scope and complexity of the cervical cancer burden and the impossibility of evidence-based decision making for health policy in a country with minimal disease-specific data and a growing disease burden. Unknowns included the prevalence of hrHPV by type, location, and age of patients; rates of under- and overdiagnosis by Pap testing for pre- and invasive cancer; number of women screened annually by Pap and their history over time; and total mortality from cervical cancer annually and over time.

In 2014 the Honduran secretary of health attempted to evaluate costs and benefits of a proposed HPV vaccine initiative for Honduras. The subsequent findings by Aguilar et al. (8) detailed their use of the London School of Hygiene and Pan American Health Organization's CERVIVAC model for the cost-effectiveness analysis. However, lack of in-country data required that many values in the algorithm be estimated or replaced with data from other (similar but not the same) countries. A key assumption in their analysis was that 70 percent of the Honduran cervical cancer is caused by hrHPV types 16 and 18, which are covered by commercially available vaccines. At that time, there was no country-specific analysis of hrHPV by type, no cancer registry, and a challenging geography that includes steep mountains and crowded urban areas. Safety is also an issue, and concerns about personal security limit people's ability to travel within the country. San Pedro Sula, the country's second largest city, is known as "the murder capital of the world." The paucity of country-specific data hampered the ability to make evidence-based recommendations to policy makers.

The enormity of the research gaps was obvious, but in order for NCCC to set up research operations in Honduras, an infrastructure had to be created. The obvious choice was to partner with existing in-country research teams. However, while eager to gain new knowledge and be part of the solution, few Honduran physicians had had the opportunity to be active in research. Clearly NCCC needed to cultivate new relationships. On a positive note, the benefits of working in a small country were immediately noticeable. The "intelligentsia" is closely connected, introductions were quickly facilitated, and acquaintances became colleagues. Everyone was eager to help stem the growing cervical cancer burden. The disease had reached all corners of the country, and for many this was personal.

The team from NCCC formed a partnership with La Liga Contra el Cancer (The League Against Cancer [LCC]), the country's sole northwestern cancer center, located in San Pedro Sula, a city of two million with a bustling industry of "sewn goods." Oncologists in LCC reported that more than half of the women who present at their clinic with cervical cancer ultimately die, having arrived too late to benefit from curative treatment.

La Liga Contra el Cancer was consistently able to bring a "reality check" to the partnership's discussions based on experience in its active hospital, where patients are treated with all types of cancer using chemotherapy, radiation therapy, and surgery. In addition to standard hospital wards, LCC offers a small communal living facility with eight beds and a stocked pantry for poor women from outside the city who are having daily treatment. At the facility, patients cook their own food and take care of each other during treatment.

Both NCCC and LCC were unsure how a partnership would progress but agreed that the focus of the research partnership would be prevention and early screening. Together, NCCC and LCC would devise and test ways to screen large numbers of women and identify the high-risk individuals.

They recognized that there would never be a sufficient number of physicians to treat the increasing number of Honduran women presenting with abnormal test results. At the insistence of LCC, the partners agreed not to consider visual inspection with ascetic acid (VIA) an option for Honduras. In the most remote global locations, VIA may be a significant improvement over no screening, but in Honduras, where every woman lives within a four- to five-hour bus ride from a treating hospital, the Hondurans decided that the standard test for screening should be the Pap test.

In an ambitious effort to screen thousands of Honduran women for cervical cancer, LCC partnered in 2011 with Universidad Catolica de Honduras (UNICAH), the largest private university in Honduras, which has a medical school in San Pedro Sula. The Program of Education and Screening in Cancer (PESCA) was founded. It is a volunteer cadre of UNICAH medical students trained in correct procedures to obtain viable cervical specimens for Pap testing by LCC pathologists. Though there is no countrywide screening or cancer registry, LCC has a valuable hospital-specific registry. PESCA became a highly significant human resource for the NCCC-LCC research partnership.

With LCC leadership and supervision, PESCA performs outreach screening at a broad variety of community-based sites for cervical cancer on weekends. At the outset, their dedication, professionalism, and ability to correctly collect specimens made them an outstanding resource. Beyond that, their experience in staffing very large outreach clinics where each *pescadore* could screen seventy or more patients per day demonstrated their ability to operationalize high-throughput, brigade-style screening. From 2010 to 2015, LCC and PESCA screened 23,670 women in the San Pedro Sula region using Pap testing.

La Jornada

Another partnership was formed with ACTS Honduras, a US-based nongovernmental organization (NGO) dedicated to community building in the Locomapa region of Honduras. This relationship provided NCCC the opportunity to leverage introductions and connections with ACTS Honduras and Honduran village leaders (HVLs). Leveraging the ACTS Honduras infrastructure, including the functioning yet rudimentary primary care clinic it supports, provided NCCC with an operational base from which to begin planning. In 2012 NCCC discussed the idea of cervical cancer screening with the HVLs and the possibility of locating a clinical trial in their village. Their reception was warm and enthusiastic. To them, a diagnosis of cancer was equivalent to a death sentence, and an opportunity to bring free screening to hundreds of women was beyond their imagination. After hearing that the goal was to operationalize the trials in a partnership that included the HVLs and would certainly require significant effort on their part, the president of the village "health and development committee" (H&D) said, "It would be an honor to be able to benefit women's health." In a key moment of sharing ownership for the program, NCCC asked the H&D to name the study, and after a half hour of debate they returned their answer: La Gran Jornada 2013. "Jornada" has no direct translation per se, but was translated to mean "large-clinical-education-event."

Midway through the planning process, NCCC and LCC decided to expand the program beyond cervical screening in recognition of the unique opportunity that would bring hundreds of women, medical personnel, and eager volunteers together at a dedicated location for a weekend of cancer screening. In what was to become typical NCCC-LCC "seize the opportunity" fashion, they added a three-part breast screening module. Women were invited to participate in a breast screening education program to learn how to examine their own breasts. An active learning module that teaches breast self-examination included practicing on standard breast models. Posters designed by WorldwideBreastCancer.org provided visual illustrations of breast abnormality. Any woman who had concerns about her breasts would be examined by an oncologist on-site. Further follow-up with imaging, if recommended by the oncologist, was to be performed at LCC.

The local H&D committee's strategy to accommodate La Gran Jornada 2013 used a variety of spaces, including classrooms and the clinic. Ultimately they recruited and scheduled volunteers, provided housing for the PESCA students, and made sure that everyone was well fed.

NCCC also relied on the HVLs to spread the word about the screening opportunity in an environment in which there are no bulletin boards, no newspapers, no television, and no Internet. About half of the village communities do not have electricity or running water in their homes. None have indoor plumbing. Person-to-person communication is the norm. One HVL became the central communicator because she had a working telephone at her house. A lifelong resident, she knew influential people in the other villages and made telephone calls or personal visits to each location to share news of the screening opportunity. This resulted in "preregistration" of 400 women from more than thirty surrounding village communities that ranged in population from 70 to 500 residents.

The H&D and LCC provided NCCC with essential information about potential and typical barriers to screening. Together with NCCC, their discussion focused on ways to mitigate the barriers. In some instances the barriers were formidable. Travel in the mountains and rural valleys is difficult and often must be negotiated on foot. There is a repurposed school bus that circulates among a dozen villages twice daily, but the fare is expensive. To maximize access to La Jornada 2013, NCCC provided a free bus that circulated from distant village communities to the screening location.

Comprehensive preparation was essential and required trust in the HVLS to execute the program as planned. In this key area, the longtime ACTS Honduras relationships proved to be valuable in bringing the right people to the table to have open and honest discussions about how to operationalize the plan. For example, each screener would need a temporary cubicle for an exam room. This was thought to be an easy requirement to meet that could be accomplished by hanging sheets to separate spaces into private cubicles. However, there was nothing to hang them from and no lumber for sale in the vicinity. Two local men went into the forest and cut down trees, hauled them out (by hand), cut the wood with a machete, and built the frames. While this solved this particular problem, another issue proved to be a challenge. Gynecological exam tables were needed. The resolution was that the tables would be designed for the screening and then, by removing the stirrups, repurposed as desks in the local school. At each roadblock, the HVLS listened carefully to understand the issue and then consulted among themselves about who to involve and how to operationalize a solution.

Two weeks before the scheduled date of Jornada 2013, when preregistration soared from 200 to 400, a second bus was added. To eliminate the economic barrier to participation, the screening itself was advertised as free. To improve a participant's comfort with the program, all frontline staff were Honduran and communicated in Spanish. The H&D rejected NCCC's suggestions that they save time by providing store-bought cookies for refreshments. Instead local women known for their cooking prepared their village's signature version of arroz con pollo for 500 diners over two days.

Jornada 2016

The relationship infrastructure continued to grow over time, and in 2015 planning for a subsequent and more complex Jornada 2016 began. The program's research goals were readjusted to reflect scientific progress and updated research questions posed by NCCC investigators and LCC oncologists. The most ambitious addition was new technology to rapidly test a large number of cervical samples for all types of hrHPV. To operationalize the technology, NCCC needed space for a "lab" to do on-site testing. Electricity in Honduras is sometimes available and sometimes not. Uneven electricity or no power at all was a legitimate concern, and NCCC talked with the HVLS about what could be a research-limiting factor. Again, local "know how" and "know who" proved vital. "No problemo," said the HVL, "I know the guy who is in charge of all the electricity for the region. I'll explain we need steady power and he'll help us out." No problem, indeed. The power stayed on for the duration of La Jornada 2016.

Planning for crowd management was a key operational focus, with hundreds of participants as the Jornada spread across the village in five separate facilities up to a quarter mile apart. Again, the existing ACTS Honduras relationships were essential, and NCCC secured the participation of Fuerza para el Futuro (Force for the Future), a local teen leadership program that is facilitated annually by ACTS Honduras to teach HVL-identified leadership skills, promote the ethic of volunteerism, and create a network of teens among many remote villages. Once the call went out, a dozen Fuerza teens in their organizational T-shirts reported for duty at 6:30 a.m. and managed all of the checkpoints and way-finding. They reveled in their official positions, holding clipboards, sporting ball caps with anticancer slogans, and handling the responsibility to check and double-check study ID numbers and control the waiting lines. Their involvement in a large and important public health program promoted youth empowerment and provided the teens with the opportunity to meet the standards for a very specific job much different from their typical daily tasks. It also served to help educate them about the importance of cervical cancer screening.

Urban Screening: Our Experience

On a parallel course to La Jornada 2016, NCCC was building infrastructure at a large factory in San Pedro Sula that employed more than 7,000 workers,

65 percent of whom were female. The factory is part of the formal economy in Honduras and thus connected with the Social Security Institute (IHSS), which provides an income tax–funded on-site infirmary. Factory workers typically see the clinician at the free infirmary for colds, cuts, and prenatal checkups. They do not use the infirmary for cancer screening. At an introductory meeting, at which NCCC and LCC described the Honduran cervical cancer burden and their new screening protocol, factory management invited NCCC to consider use of their physical plant as a location for a screening trial.

In addition to the factory's workforce of 4,550 females, the factory is part of the citywide Maquila Association, which represents many factories employing more than 250,000 women. The factory agreed to commit space, cooperation from management, and access to in-house communications channels, including bulletin boards and overhead announcements. Worktime entertainer DJ King Kong, who plays music during work shifts, would also provide commentary intended to educate workers about the screening program.

A decision was made in late 2015 to mount two cancer screening clinical trials in April 2016 utilizing NCCC's infrastructure in the villages and at the factory. A memorandum of understanding between NCCC and LCC and another between NCCC and the committee of HVL were signed. The two screenings in 2016 were planned for dissimilar locations—La Jornada in the rural village and the other in the urban factory—but both would test for hrHPV. Most important was the team's decision to "meet women where they are." In a cost-effectiveness framework, Campos encouraged decision makers who were grappling with challenges of scaling up cervical screening to develop evidence-based protocols to maximize health benefits under operational constraints. (11) The partners were interested in the same goals: to get the test results to the women quickly to minimize loss to follow-up, build in-country capacity for future research partnerships, mitigate local barriers to participation, and analyze the data for policy making.

The two locations were dissimilar in ways the team recognized from the start: urban and rural, more and less educated, and a tighter group agewise in the factory versus a broader age range in the village. A difference they had not accounted for was the perception of time. In a factory, time is money, and a tight schedule with rapid throughput to minimize time away from the sewing machines was essential to preserving management backing. Conversely, in the village the pace is slower, and social customs such as a pleasant lunch and a well-paced greeting are valued. These differences make the comparison of approaches interesting and potentially useful to others planning outreach screening. NCCC's long-term goal was to develop a portable screening protocol that could be scaled up and sustained in other countries and situations. Accordingly, it limited site or culturally specific modifications to make the protocol as adaptable as possible without exceptional efforts or infrastructure.

The 400 participants for hrHPV screening were recruited by simple flyers on the factory's bulletin boards and doors. Female employees of all ages were invited to be screened. An information table was set up near the restroom and staffed by LCC and PESCA staff. Women could come and ask questions about the study and complete a preconsent process. The response rate was fantastic. Accrual of 400 participants was rapid and completed by noon on the second day. Factory management provided a room, usually used for meetings, that was adapted for the mini-screening clinic. At just thirteen square meters with three exam cubicles fashioned from simple lumber and curtains, the mini-clinic was a tight fit for the necessary supplies (including speculums, slides, cyto-brushes, and exam gloves); a registration desk for the final consent process; and the laboratory desk that held the PCR instrument, study laptop computer, and setup to extract DNA. At the registration desk, each participant was assigned a study ID number, and all study data were stored securely in "the cloud."

According to plan, PESCA volunteers staffing the screening cubicles for the ten-day study were supervised by an LCC physician. An LCC pathologist, trained at NCCC in New Hampshire, staffed the lab desk, with backup consultation by telephone and e-mail as necessary with NCCC personnel. Factory management contributed an executive assistant who ultimately staffed the registration table for the duration of the study. Her ability to connect quickly with factory personnel from custodians to the management proved to be an essential resource.

For each woman's screening, the PESCA inserted a speculum and used cyto-brushes (preferred by NCCC) to obtain three cervical specimens from each participant. The first specimen was the source of DNA extracted for the hrHPV testing. If a woman was hrHPV positive, her second specimen was used for a traditional Pap smear test to determine the presence of pre- or invasive cervical cancer. The third specimen was reserved for evaluation at NCCC laboratories to check for concordance between the PCR assay used in Honduras at the factory and established laboratory standards. Each participant received a letter with her results via the factory's in-house mail system for employees. There is no functional postal system in Honduras. Most women had some literacy, and those unable to read their letters asked others for assistance; this is common in Honduras. Women with positive Pap smear tests received letters from LCC explaining the results and encouraging them to make an appointment soon for clinical follow-up.

NCCC's expectations of accuracy plus rapid throughput required close attention to the protocol. LCC's management perspective was essential in resolving any situations that slowed throughput. The data show a remarkable screening rate of just five to eight minutes per participant. Screening for all 400 participants was completed in 7.5 days.

Post-study, participants and nonparticipants commented in a facilitated focus group about their experience. Overall, they considered the free screening at their workplace to be a tremendous benefit, particularly because of the convenience. They were less positive about the catcalls and negative comments from male coworkers when women left their workstations to attend the screening clinic.

Oncologists at LCC reported that only half of the women who received letters encouraging clinical follow-up because of positive Pap tests complied without prompting. Women who did not respond were reminded to do so by calls to their mobile phones. The on-site physician working at the infirmary talked to the final few who had not complied. Most who did not comply said they were busy working and could not be excused from work. In fact, the factory had a policy of no loss of pay for excusable absences because of medical appointments; however, the women were unaware of the policy and the mechanism to use it. When informed of the mechanism, all of the formerly noncompliant women followed through with clinical appointments. For the five women who tested hrHPV positive, subsequent colposcopies showed that three had preinvasive cancer, and two were diagnosed with invasive cancer. All were treated by loop electrosurgical excision procedure (LEEP) at LCC and will be followed over time.

After the factory screening project, the Jornada 2016 project was held in the selected rural village community. Residents of the Locomapa region of Honduras live more than three hours from any city. The dirt road can be impassable due to washouts, and many of the rural village communities are an hour or more walking distance from a road of any type. Virtually all residents are part of subsistence farming families; some have very limited income from the sale of agricultural products such as corn, beans, or livestock. Other families, typically indigenous people, manufacture lump charcoal. Access to primary care is through small government health units, each staffed by a recent medical graduate who is required to do a year of social service in the outpost. Supplies of medications are severely limited or they are unavailable, and there is no cancer screening.

Jornada 2016 was scheduled for a Saturday and Sunday; the 2013 Jornada's person-to-person marketing plan was reused but augmented by colorful posters displayed in the closest cluster of twelve village communities. The study accrued its limit of 400 women from forty village communities. Any woman over age eighteen, regardless of her home village community, was welcome to participate in the Jornada. Dozens more who arrived after the study registration was closed were tested for cervical cancer by Pap only and connected with follow-up care as appropriate.

After Jornada 2013, NCCC and LCC had realized that an open invitation made any useful measurement of participation rates impossible. Government census statistics were not granular enough to yield information to the level of "women of screening age" (between eighteen and seventy years old), so just a few days after Jornada 2016, the team took the unusual step of commissioning a site-specific census. The focus was the cluster of twelve village communities, and HVLs were instructed to count the women of screening age in each of the twelve locations. For the purposes of the study, the count was to include any women, whether regular residents or visitors, sleeping in the village that weekend who were over age eighteen and not elderly, which was defined in that area by infirmity, not a specific age. Locally, the elderly do not travel from their homes, so their participation would be unrealistic. Participation rates for the cluster of twelve village communities ranged from 5 to 84 percent.

Given that all twelve communities received the same posters with Jornada 2016 information as well as the telephone or person-to-person marketing by the HVLs, the great difference in participation rates merited further investigation. Investigators wondered if there had been a bad experience in 2013 that made women choose not to participate in 2016. Perhaps no one in their community had been found to have pre- or invasive cancer in 2013 and it was deemed not worth the time and effort to participate again. Another possibility was a competing community event, such as a wedding or funeral scheduled for the same time. To investigate, two female Honduran team members from LCC visited the village communities that had low participation rates about three months after Jornada 2016, to ask: Did they know about the Jornada? Did they participate? How could the Jornada be improved?

In the course of those informal interviews, women uniformly praised the Jornada model, reported being well informed about the opportunity, and had a variety of reasons if they did not participate. These included having "heard" that a cutoff of 400 participants had been reached and being unable to catch the free bus because of personal activities. For the future, Jornada marketing will make it clear that all women who arrive before the published ending time will be screened for cancer, regardless of whether they are accrued to a study.

Operationalizing the Jornada in 2013 was challenging because it was a novel activity, the number of participants was unpredictable, and though eager, the local volunteers were untested in this setting. In 2016, buoyed by the smooth operation of the 2013 Jornada, the NCCC-LCC partnership was emboldened to increase the screening activities from breast and cervical cancer to also include thyroid cancer. LCC had perceived thyroid cancer as significantly increased in its clinics, particularly among young women presenting with late-stage disease. Screening for oral cancer was also included. These cancers are highly prevalent in Honduras and could be tested on-site and treated at LCC.

The next challenge was setting up the flow of Jornada 2016 so that participants would be as comfortable as possible throughout the several-hour process and perceive their experience as organized and professional. Women traveled to the Jornada 2016 site as before: by the free bus, on foot, on the back of a motor-scooter driven by a male family member, or on horseback. They dressed very nicely; unbeknown to the NCCC and LCC planners, the HVLs told other village leaders: "This is a formal occasion. Women should bathe and wear their nice clothes." To reduce confusion, women were asked not to bring children unless they were babes in arms. They brought their Honduran identification cards, which became the "identifiable" numbers linked only by an IRB-approved "data crosswalk" to their newly assigned and "de-identified" study identification numbers.

The women's first step in the study process, located in an elementary school classroom, was the registration and consent process. To demystify the consent process and accommodate nonreaders, groups of ten were gathered for the informative part of the consent process and then each prospective participant was afforded an individual interview with a registrar, who also administered the study registration and intake survey. LCC staff were prepared with felt-tip pens to color the women's fingertips in case a fingerprint was needed in lieu of a signature. Data from the survey and comparison of study rosters from 2013 and 2016 revealed that about half of the women were study participants at both Jornadas. Once registered and having consented, participants were provided with zipped plastic bags containing study materials, including cyto-brushes, labels with their study IDs, and their registration surveys. In the research scheme, each participant would transport her own records from activity to activity. Completed consent forms were retained at the central registration area.

The second screening was set in the local medical-dental clinic, which was a ten-minute walk from the elementary school. Eight cubicles were constructed of locally harvested lumber, and the gynecological exam tables used in Jornada 2013 were retrieved from their repurposed use as classroom desks. In this location, the PESCA screeners called participants, who were waiting in line in the shade, one at a time into their cubicles. Women exiting from the clinic were generous in their encouragement to those who were waiting, saying, "It didn't hurt at all" or "Don't be scared."

Tucked into the clinic, where every cubic inch was prioritized, were an active primary care exam room and the laboratory. At Jornada 2013, approximately 10 percent of participants had a medical complaint of enough significance to warrant immediate referral to primary care. Less urgent complaints were referred to the regular weekday clinic. Screeners in 2016 found the same rate of complaints needing immediate attention from a primary care clinician. The modest laboratory consisted of a countertop, a cold water sink, a folding table, an overhead light, a fan, and several chairs. It was fitted with the PCR instrument, equipment for extracting DNA from the cervical samples, and a laptop study computer.

In the cubicles the screeners followed the identical protocol that had been established for the factory project. Three cervical samples were taken. The first was used for PCR typing for hrHPV, the second was forwarded for Pap testing if the initial sample was positive for hrHPV, and the third sample was forwarded to NCCC for concordance testing. The screeners time-stamped the registration forms when the women were ushered into the cubicles and when the exam was completed.

Screening for thyroid cancer by manual palpation and for oral cancer by visual scan was conducted in the kindergarten classroom. In the case of visible oral lesions, the screener used a dental camera to image the lesions for later review via telepathology at NCCC. Locomapa residents have had no access to professional dentistry and have to resort to care from a "construction dentist," who is essentially a man with a set of pliers. Understandably, the screener found decayed teeth and lesions and reported many participants in pain. One thyroid cancer was suspected and later identified by biopsy at LCC as cancer. The thyroid screener also identified five goiters.

Breast education and screening were conducted in the school library. The setup included six round tables with chairs, a tall vinyl poster describing the breast self-exam technique, eight brown-skinned standard breast models with embedded "lumps," and copies of the Worldwidebreastcancer.org "lemons" egg-crate graphic that illustrates numerous different external signs of breast problems. Women rotated into the breast activity area and joined tables with other women to follow along with the PESCA instructors, who presented the breast self-exam instructions. The instructors, trained by LCC, were all male and had been assigned the task because LCC had previously observed that women tend to pay more attention if the demonstration, given with a hand under the presenter's own shirt, is delivered by a man. Nervous giggling was common, and the presenters sometimes interrupted their instructions to admonish the women to pay attention, saying, "This is important, please pay attention." Shortly after one of those moments, a woman found an area of concern in her own breast and the mood became very sober.

All women participated in the education and then were split into two groups dependent on whether they were lactating or not. The lactating group was relocated to another venue for educational videos on breast-feeding. The nonlactating group was offered access to the clinical breast exam. In each of the 2013 and 2016 Jornadas, more than a dozen women were referred to LCC for imaging of suspicious masses.

Finally, participants walked to the community center, where their plastic bags with registration data and activity time-stamps were collected and exchanged for token gifts in thanks for their participation. They joined the participants on the lactation track in watching health education videos, were served an arroz con pollo luncheon, and chatted while waiting for the bus to take them home.

Implementation of Local hrHPV Screening:
The Challenges

Cervical cancer screening in LMICs encounters numerous challenges that are not typical in the high-income countries. While Pap smear testing is a routine occurrence for those women who have access to clinical care, the more advanced liquid cytology Pap test is not available. In addition to traditional Pap smears having technological limitations, there is the burden of not having enough trained pathologists to read the slides.

NCCC's implementation of a novel screening protocol including selection and validation of an hrHPV test and instrument for hrHPV detection that would be portable and require minimum maintenance was a challenge. The test needed to be robust and able to perform in extreme environmental conditions without refrigeration for reagent storage. NCCC designed a method for DNA extraction from cervical swab specimens that was crude yet produced quality DNA to use in the hrHPV test. The simple extraction process used a boiling water bath for isolation of DNA, and lyophilized reagents that could be stored at room temperature were used in a real-time PCR with a semi-portable SLAN system.

NCCC opted to introduce hrHPV screening using molecular methods to help alleviate the need for Pap smear testing and slide reading for every woman while also providing a more advanced and sensitive test. Implementation of such technology in a resource-limited setting included its own challenges. Most clinical staff in Honduras had never performed laboratory techniques before, and definitely not techniques such as pipetting, which is a core skill in molecular pathology. This was addressed by a one-week intensive training session at NCCC for two Honduran pathologists.

To make significant inroads in preventing cervical cancer in LMICs, widespread effective screening must be convenient for women. The goal of meeting women where they are requires innovative collaborations, stable infrastructure, and robust technology for excellence in testing. In LMICs, where pathology staff and facilities are often overburdened and under-resourced, the challenge is to develop and promote screening protocols that maximize local human resources in pathology by utilizing better screening technology. PCR screening for hrHPV, followed by Pap testing only for women who are hrHPV positive, facilitates amplification of each pathologist's throughput. Prescreening for hrHPV reduces the percent of the population to be Pap tested, allowing a tremendous increase in the total number of women screened without increasing the burden on pathology services.

Local barriers to screening can include fear of cancer, language differences, long turnaround time for test results, poor connection to clinical follow-up, lack of knowledge about screening, distance to screening, no social support for screening, and costs. By working closely with Hondurans, the NCCC research and screening team was able to mitigate barriers and successfully attract women to participate in cancer screening.

In the factory setting, the key was convenience for women. As busy working women with families who rely on public transportation, the opportunity to take an important step toward preventing cancer while at the worksite was of great value. To this group of women, time and convenience were paramount. The rural women living in small villages placed a priority on value and the opportunity for free screening. As subsistence farmers in a remote location, there is very little cash in their local economy, and paying for screening is not a viable option.

The Jornada model, which was heavily reliant on PESCA, demonstrated the ability of well-trained medical students to obtain cervical specimens in an efficient, effective, and professional manner. Informal conversations among women, overheard in the factory and the village, often included comments about the students' professionalism and kindness. At the other end of their involvement, more than 99 percent of the specimens they obtained contained sufficient DNA to perform the extraction necessary for testing by PCR.

The importance of field-testing both technology and tactics in an LMIC cannot be overstated. Laboratory testing confirms efficacy, but significant field-testing determines effectiveness. In biomedical testing, the measure of excellence is a result of both high sensitivity, which is the ability to accurately identify people with a disease, and high specificity, which is the ability to accurately identify people without a disease. To eventually translate new science from laboratory settings for use into practical solutions or recommendations that will prevent or reduce the cancer burden in LMICs, investigators must commit to field-testing hypotheses in situations that often are unpredictable and difficult.

Sustainability is important. Screening programs are expensive, and finding sufficient funding to maintain them is always a challenge. Funding for these screening studies was provided by NCCC and a Munck-Pfefferkorn translational research grant from Dartmouth's Geisel School of Medicine.

Conclusion

Our experience working for and promoting women's health in an LMIC highlights several critical features necessary to allow for successful clinical implementation, translational research, and sustainability. Key to these successes have been the grassroots relationships among investigators, local clinicians, and village residents. Working in a true partnership model of community-led research allows for inclusion of all parties in the design and implementation of studies that will benefit all involved. Our work in Honduras has led to lifelong relationships with colleagues and individuals clearly impacted by these efforts. We collectively have created the groundwork for sustained hrHPV screening and efforts that will lead to future Jornadas and hopefully to a pathway that will reduce cervical cancer mortality among Honduran women.

References

1. Rural poverty portal [cited 2016 Oct 27]. Available from: www.ruralpoverty portal.org/country/home/tags/HN.

2. Pasquali V. The poorest countries in the world. Global Fin Mag 2017 Feb 13 [cited 2017 Sep 1] Available from: https://www.gfmag.com/global-data/economic-data/the -poorest-countries-in-the-world?page=12.

3. UNICEF information by country: Honduras [cited 2016 Oct 27]. Available from: www.unicef.org/country/hnd.

4. Sankarayaranana R. Screening for cancer in low- and middle-income countries. Ann Global Health 2014;80:412–7.

5. Bejarano S. Personal interview with Linda Kennedy [electronic mail]. 2016 Sep 14.

6. Cerrato J. (Honduran Institute of Social Security). Personal interview with Linda Kennedy. 2016 Aug 1.

7. Perkins RB, Langrish S, Stern LJ, et al. A community-based education program about cervical cancer improves knowledge and screening behavior in Honduran women. Rev Panam Salud Publica 2007;22(3):187–93.

8. Aguilar IBM, Mendoza LO, Garcia O, et al. Cost effectiveness analysis of the introduction of the human papilloma vaccine in Honduras. Vaccine 2015;33(Suppl 1): A167–73.

9. Caterino R, Petignat P, Dongui l, et al. Cervical cancer screening in developing countries at a crossroad: emerging technologies and policy choices. World J Clin Oncol 2015;6(6):281–90.

10. Denny L. Screening for cervical cancer in resource-limited settings. UpToDate. Wolters Kluwer [cited 2016 Sep 14]. Available from: https://www.uptodate.com /contents/screening-for-cervical-cancer-in-resource-limited-settings.

11. Campos NG, Castle PE, Wright TC, et al. Cervical cancer screening in low-resource settings: a cost-effectiveness framework for valuing tradeoffs between test performance and program coverage. Int J Cancer 2015;137(9):2208–19.

Chapter 8

A. Ross Kerr, Shelly Arora, and Paul M. Speight

Oral Cancer Screening in Low- and Middle-Income Countries

Introduction

Cancer Screening: An Overview

Cancer screening is defined as the application of a simple and cost-effective test to a large population of patients who are asymptomatic and apparently free of cancer in order to identify those who may have cancer. (1) A screening test is not a diagnostic test; it is intended to identify tissue changes that may indicate the likelihood of someone having or developing cancer. A positive screening test is then confirmed by further diagnostic testing to identify the presence or absence of cancer. Screening encompasses a process of testing and then referring those who test positive for definitive diagnosis. Screening programs target a defined population (general population or high-risk population). They can be managed by either a regional or a national program, or in opportunistic settings. Screenings for cervical, breast, and colorectal cancer are well-known examples of programs that have been implemented in many countries.

With few exceptions, the burden of cancer is disproportionally greater in low- and middle-income countries (LMICs) than in high-income countries. The stratification of countries by income is based on the World Bank country group classifications, as defined by 2013 per capita gross national monthly income: low-income countries (less than US$1,045), lower middle-income countries (US$1,046 to US$4,125), and upper middle-income countries (US$4,126 to US$12,745). (2)

Criteria for Cancer Screening Programs

Not all cancers are amenable to screening, and consideration of a screening program must be based on meeting a number of essential criteria to ensure maximum public health gains in a cost-effective manner. As an example, in the United Kingdom the National Screening Committee examines twenty criteria before a screening program may be funded and implemented. (3) (See table 8.1.) In the United States the US Preventive Services Task Force provides methodology for the development of recommendations for screening and other preventive services. (4) In LMICs the processes for implementation for cancer screening, if any, are part of a World Health Organization (WHO) cancer control plan. (5)

The suitability of a specific cancer for population-based screening must be determined by a clear understanding of the natural history of the disease. Some cancers, such as cervical and colorectal cancer, have a long natural history characterized by asymptomatic "precancerous" lesions, a predictable proportion of which undergo malignant transformation over a specified period of time. Screening that identifies patients with such precancerous changes should result in treatment that should lead to an increase in survival. (See chapter 2.) The natural history of other cancers, such as breast cancer, may not be as predictable, and screening may be based on data demonstrating a benefit to detecting early-stage cancers; screening programs for such cancers should lead to improvements in morbidity and reduction in mortality.

Cancer burden also dictates the type of screening approach applied. Countries with a high burden of advanced-stage cancer are more likely to focus resources on screening programs geared toward early detection and down-staging the cancer. This chapter focuses on the feasibility of screening for oral cancer, a cancer that generally has a poor prognosis and is highly prevalent in many LMICs.

Oral Cancer and Oral Potentially Malignant Disorders

Oral cancer comprises a subset of head and neck cancers and is often loosely defined as cancer involving the oral cavity and the oropharynx. More than 90 percent arise from the epithelial lining as squamous cell carcinomas. Oral cavity cancers are distinct from lip and oropharyngeal cancers

Table 8.1. UK Government Guidance on Criteria for the Implementation of a Screening Program

The Condition

1. The condition should be an important health problem, as determined by its frequency and/or severity. The epidemiology, incidence, prevalence, and natural history of the condition should be understood, including development from latent to declared disease, and/or there should be robust evidence about the association between the risk or disease marker and serious or treatable disease.
2. All the cost-effective, primary prevention interventions should have been implemented as far as practicable.
3. If the carriers of a mutation are identified as a result of screening, the natural history of people with this status should be understood, including the psychological implications.

The Test

4. There should be a simple, safe, precise, and validated screening test.
5. The distribution of test values in the target population should be known and a suitable cutoff level defined and agreed upon.
6. The test, from sample collection to delivery of results, should be acceptable to the target population.
7. There should be an agreed upon policy on the further diagnostic investigation of individuals with a positive test result and on the choices available to those individuals.
8. If the test is for a particular mutation or set of genetic variants, the method for their selection and the means through which these will be kept under review in the program should be clearly set out.

The Treatment

9. There should be an effective intervention for patients identified through screening, with evidence that intervention at a pre-symptomatic phase leads to better outcomes for the screened individual than usual care. Evidence relating to wider benefits of screening, for example those relating to family members, should be taken into account where available. However, where there is no prospect of benefit for the individual screened, the screening program shouldn't be further considered.
10. There should be agreed upon, evidence-based policies covering which individuals should be offered intervention and the appropriate intervention to be offered.

Table 8.1. (*continued*)

The Screening Program

11. There should be evidence from high-quality, randomized, controlled trials that the screening program is effective in reducing mortality or morbidity. Where screening is aimed solely at providing information to allow the person being screened to make an "informed choice," there must be evidence from high-quality trials that the test accurately measures risk. The information that is provided about the test and its outcome must be of value and readily understood by the individual being screened.
12. There should be evidence that the complete screening program (test, diagnostic procedures, treatment/intervention) is clinically, socially, and ethically acceptable to health professionals and the public.
13. The benefit gained by individuals from the screening program should outweigh any harm, for example from overdiagnosis, overtreatment, false positives, false reassurance, uncertain findings, and complications.
14. The opportunity cost of the screening program (including testing, diagnosis and treatment, administration, training, and quality assurance) should be economically balanced in relation to expenditure on medical care as a whole (value for money). Assessment against this criteria should take into consideration evidence from cost benefit and/or cost-effectiveness analyses and the effective use of available resources.

Implementation Criteria

15. Clinical management of the condition and patient outcomes should be optimized in all health care providers prior to participation in a screening program.
16. All other options for managing the condition should have been considered (such as improving treatment or providing other services), to ensure that no more cost-effective intervention could be introduced or current interventions increased within the resources available.
17. There should be a plan for managing and monitoring the screening program and an agreed upon set of quality assurance standards.
18. Adequate staffing and facilities for testing, diagnosis, treatment, and program management should be available prior to the commencement of the screening program.
19. Evidence-based information, explaining the purpose and potential consequences of screening, investigation, and preventative intervention or treatment, should be made available to potential participants to assist them in making an informed choice.
20. Public pressure for widening the eligibility criteria for reducing the screening interval and for increasing the sensitivity of the testing process should be anticipated. Decisions about these parameters should be scientifically justifiable to the public.

in terms of etiopathogenesis, prognosis, and management. Lip cancer is strongly associated with ultraviolet light exposure; oral cavity cancer is typically associated with risk factors such as tobacco, areca nut, and heavy alcohol use. Oropharyngeal cancer is largely associated with human papillomavirus (HPV) infection. For the purposes of this chapter we define oral cancer as cancer involving oral cavity subsites (International Classification of Diseases coding system, ICD-10 C02-C06).

Definition

Oral potentially malignant disorders (OPMDs) comprise a subset of oral epithelial lesions encountered clinically that may represent either a malignancy or a "precancerous" lesion with a higher risk of becoming malignant over time. The most common OPMDs are leukoplakia and erythroplakia (or mixed lesions known as erythroleukoplakia). Leukoplakia is defined herein as white plaques of questionable risk having excluded (other) known diseases or disorders that carry no increased risk for cancer, and erythroplakia is defined as a fiery red patch that cannot be characterized clinically or pathologically as any other definable disease. (6) Oral submucous fibrosis is another OPMD, associated with areca nut use, and carries a risk for malignant transformation. (7)

Global Epidemiology of Oral Cancer/OPMDs

Global epidemiologic data for oral cancer are updated annually by the WHO. It is challenging to obtain a full picture of the epidemiology of oral cancer because cancer registries for many LMICs may not capture data that are truly representative of the general population. Further, registries have traditionally grouped lip, oral cavity, and pharyngeal sites as the single entity "oral cancer." That being said, the International Agency for Research on Cancer's (IARC's) GLOBOCAN 2012 reported that oral cavity cancer (defined as ICD-10 C00-08 sites) is among the most common cancers worldwide, with a collective incidence estimated to be 300,000 new cases per annum with 145,400 deaths. There is wide variation in trends reported across the world by region, sex, age, and subsite. (8) It is noteworthy that two-thirds of oral cancer cases occur in LMICs. Despite advances in treatment, the five-year survival rate for oral cancer has remained static at about 50 percent; the most important determinant explaining these poor statistics is diagnostic delay, as more than 60 percent of patients present with advanced-stage disease (stage III/IV). (9) The primary treatment modality is surgery, with adjuvant radiation or chemo radiation for advanced disease and immuno-therapy for patients who do not respond to the conventional treatment. The morbidity of the acute and chronic sequelae of such treatments, particularly of radiation, has a significant impact on the quality of life of oral cancer patients. These treatment modalities are also very costly, usually out of the reach of many cancer patients living in LMICS.

The majority of oral cancers are preceded by OPMDS, although unlike cervical neoplasia, the natural history of OPMDS and malignant transforma-tion does not always follow a linear path and can be difficult to predict. (10) Leukoplakia has an estimated global prevalence of 2.6 percent (95% CI: 1.72–2.74%) (11), and the overall malignant transformation rate is estimated to be < 5 percent, although this may vary considerably according to the clinical phenotype of the lesion and the presence or degree of epithelial dysplasia. (12) The major risk factors for oral cancer and OPMDS are tobacco (smoked and chewed), areca nut chewing, and high alcohol consumption. (13)

Oral Cancer Screening

The phrase "oral cancer screening" has been used imprecisely in the litera-ture to describe the process of detecting oral malignancies and/or OPMDS in various clinical settings such as the dental office. Oral cancer screening in the strictest sense is defined as the organized application of an oral cancer screening test to a large population who are asymptomatic and apparently free of cancer in order to identify those who may have oral cancer. Such "organized" screening is distinct from the typical "opportunistic" screening or "case finding" that a patient might undergo during a routine dental visit. Organized screening programs invite patients to undergo the screening and have centralized responsibility for key elements of the process, such as eligibility requirements, quality assurance, follow-up, recall, and program evaluation. Even though the actual test may be identical to that performed during an "opportunistic" screening, the test offered by a dentist or health professional involves no population oversight. (14)

Few countries have implemented national oral cancer screening pro-grams. Most oral cancer screening guidelines and/or recommendations issued by national authoritative bodies (governments or specialty organi-zations such as the American Academy of Oral Medicine) tend to be geared toward early detection by "frontline" dental providers in an opportunistic setting. (15)

This chapter attempts to provide a balanced review outlining the evidence base for the screening of oral cancer and OPMDs in LMICs, using the criteria from the UK National Screening Committee as a "gold" standard to assess whether the evidence supports oral cancer screening. The following sections follow the main headings listed in table 8.1.

Oral Cancer and OPMDs: The Condition

In terms of "the condition," the significant global burden of oral cancer (particularly in LMICs) demonstrates that this is an important health problem with significant mortality and morbidity. The natural history suggests that most oral cancers are preceded by an OPMD. However, there is some uncertainty about the inevitability and timeline for progression and malignant transformation. Clinical features of OPMDs coupled with histopathology can provide insight into the natural history, although there are currently no commercially available, validated biomarkers that can predict with high accuracy which OPMDs or patients with such lesions will undergo malignant transformation. (16) For this reason, oral cancer generally meets criterion 1. In terms of criterion 2, programs have been implemented for the primary prevention of the established risk factors of oral cancer, particularly the control of tobacco. Low- and middle-income countries, however, may be lagging behind high-income countries in this regard. Oral cancer has a heterogeneous mutational landscape (17) and as yet no single genetic or epigenetic alteration (or collection of alterations) has been established to suggest that criterion 3 is applicable to oral cancer.

Oral Cancer and OPMDs: The Test

The conventional oral examination (COE) is used in the majority of oral cancer screening studies. It is both simple and safe to perform; there is no sample collection; and it comprises a precise series of steps allowing a trained examiner to both visually inspect and palpate the tissues of the oral cavity and extra-oral structures, such as the regional lymph nodes, with the aim of identifying a lesion (or lesions) that carries an index of "suspicion" for oral cancer or OPMDs. The index of suspicion relates to the features of clinical presentation that satisfy criteria for the clinical diagnosis of oral cancer or OPMDs.

The validity of the COE is predicated on the frequency with which a result, whether positive or negative, is confirmed by an acceptable diagnostic procedure that determines the gold standard diagnosis. The ability of any screening test to classify as positive those persons with the disease is termed "sensitivity," (18) and the ability to classify as negative those without the disease is termed "specificity." Sensitivity is a measure of the false-negative rate and specificity of the false-positive rate. For population-based screening, an acceptable threshold for sensitivity and specificity must be considered carefully. A highly sensitive test yields a low false-negative rate and translates to fewer patients who have the disease than receive a negative test result. However, highly sensitive tests can be expensive to administer, so cost must be considered. Conversely, a highly specific test is important to reduce avoidable costs due to unnecessary diagnostic workup of false-positive results, overtreatment, and associated adverse psychological and physical effects. Almost all LMICs have limited resources. For them, national "organized" screening programs are typically more cost-effective than "opportunistic" screening.

Other test variables are the positive and negative predictive values (PPVs, NPVs). The former is the probability that subjects with a positive screening test truly have the disease, and the latter is the probability that subjects with a negative screening test truly do not have the disease. These values are of importance in the context of the prevalence of the disease. Sensitivity, specificity, PPV, and NPV determine the value of the screening test.

The validity of the conventional oral examination as a screening test for oral cancer and OMPDs in LMICs has been evaluated in numerous studies, although only five studies based on "organized" screening trials have yielded data that can provide sensitivity and specificity. (See summary in table 8.2.) The screeners performed the COE, and subjects were deemed "screen positive" (having oral cancer or OPMDs) or "screen negative" (having no lesions or lesions with no apparent malignant potential) using specified clinical criteria as defined by each study. The gold standard was either the clinical diagnosis of an OPMD (true positive) or normal (a benign diagnosis) (true negative) following referral and reexamination by a specialist, or histopathologic diagnosis, in which squamous cell carcinoma or epithelial dysplasia rendered a positive outcome.

In a Taiwanese study, the screening test reported a sensitivity and specificity of an impressive 99 percent. (19) In this study, experienced otolaryngologists and dentists performed the screenings, and the COE was compared to a histopathologic gold standard. The use of experts to perform screenings may explain the high accuracy to rule in or rule out oral cancer. Other studies conducted in Sri Lanka (20,21) and India (22,23) utilized health

Table 8.2. Reports of Evaluations of Conventional Oral Examinations from Screening Programs in LMICs (in which sensitivity and specificity of the test could be calculated)

	LMIC	No. screened	screen+ ref (%)	Gold std +	prev	SE	SP
Mehta et al. (23)	India	39,331	67	1,921	1.4	0.59	0.98
Warnakulasuriya et al. (20)	Sri Lanka	29,295	54	384	1.3	0.95	0.81
Warnakulasuriya et al. (21)	Sri Lanka	57,124	62	1,745	6.2	0.97	0.75
Mathew et al. (22)	India	2,069	NA	212	10.2	0.94	0.98
Chang et al. (19)	Taiwan	13,878	63	282	2.0	0.99	0.99

workers who had undergone intensive training to conduct the screenings. In the India study, "screen positive" subjects were referred for specialist reexamination, and in order to calculate the false-negative rate, specialists rescreened a subset of the "screen negative" subjects in the field. Three of these four studies reported a high sensitivity (94–97%), and one reported a low sensitivity of 0.59 (a 41% false-negative rate), which the authors attributed to a wide variation in the number of subjects screened by numerous health care workers who participated in the study.

There was an increasing trend in sensitivity values as health care workers gained experience by screening a larger number of subjects. In terms of specificity, of the four studies utilizing health workers, two of the studies reported high specificity (98%), and the two Sri Lankan studies reported a lower specificity (81% and 75%, respectively). This finding may be explained by the expanded criteria used for a referable "screen positive" lesion, which included some benign entities. The prevalence ranged from 1.3 to 10.1 percent. In all probability, the prevalence values were underestimates because of the large percentage of "screen positive" subjects who were not reexamined (33–46%), coupled with the inexact method for determining the false-negative rates. The PPV and NPV were not reported.

A recent systematic review analyzing studies from both high-income countries and LMICs confirmed that the COE showed very high specificity (98%), and the authors concluded that the COE was deemed to be better at correctly classifying the absence of OPMDs or oral cavity cancer in disease-free individuals than at classifying their presence in diseased individuals. (24)

Studies to validate other oral cancer screening tests, including mouth self-examination (MSE) and the use of vital staining, have been conducted. The two studies relying on MSE, one conducted in India (25) and the other in the United Kingdom (26), yielded low sensitivity (<33%) and would not be suitable as a population screening test for oral cancer or OPMDs. A well-powered, randomized, controlled trial that explored the use of a toluidine blue oral rinse as a screening adjunct to the COE was conducted in an organized population screening program. (27) A greater percentage of oral cancer and OPMDs was detected in the group undergoing COE plus toluidine blue versus COE alone, although this was not statistically significant, suggesting that the addition of vital staining is not warranted. The use of salivary and serum-based screening tests for oral cancer and OPMDs is appealing, particularly noninvasive salivary screening tests. Although there are platforms under development, no validation studies have been conducted as yet.

It is important to stress that oral cancer and OPMDs have variable clinical presentations that have been well defined and classified, although these definitions unfortunately are not always consistently applied across research studies. The distribution of positive test values, equivalent to the prevalence of the disease in a given population, is also variable. Low- and middle-income countries typically have a higher prevalence of disease, which in contrast with high-income countries with a lower disease prevalence should translate into a higher positive predictive value of a screening test. (28)

Patients who are screened as "positive" are typically referred for further diagnostic evaluation by an expert. The gold standard test to render a definitive diagnosis remains a tissue biopsy followed by histopathologic analysis to confirm or rule out malignancy (such as squamous cell carcinoma) or epithelial dysplasia. Based on the studies reported in table 8.2, a large percentage of patients who are screened as "positive" do not undergo further investigation. There are various reasons for this. (29)

Criterion 5 states that "the distribution of test values in the target population should be known and a suitable cut-off level defined and agreed." In terms of the COE, there are no "test values" on a continuous scale, but rather a dichotomous value of positive (meaning there is a lesion that meets the clinical criteria for an OPMD or oral cancer) versus negative (meaning there is no oral lesion deemed to have malignant potential).

Although studies have identified the advantages and shortcomings of a COE (see the summary in table 8.3, as adapted from Speight [30]), the data do support the validity of the COE as a screening test for oral cancer or OPMDs in LMICs when performed by well-trained and experienced health care workers. There is sufficient evidence for COE as a test to satisfy criteria 4–7. However, criterion 8 is not applicable because there are no currently available genetic tests for oral cancer or OPMDs.

Oral Cancer and OPMDs: The Treatment

There are evidence-based treatments for oral cancer (31), including surgery, radiation, chemotherapy, and immunotherapy, which have been ratified by many LMICs. (32) However, the management of patients diagnosed with OPMDs/oral epithelial dysplasia is controversial. (33) A recent systematic review of efficacy studies employing chemopreventive agents revealed no agents that have been demonstrated to reduce malignant transformation. (34) A systematic review of the surgical management of OPMDs reported that surgery reduces malignant transformation rates, although the heterogeneity of results across these nonrandomized controlled trials suggests more research is needed. (35) Evidence to support or refute close surveillance and serial biopsy of patients with OPMDs is lacking.

Given that the majority of patients who are "screen positive" do not have oral cancer (most have OPMDs, of which about 95 percent will probably not progress), there is mixed evidence that intervention at a pre-symptomatic phase leads to better outcomes for individuals with OPMDs. Based on the evidence, the conclusion is that criteria 9 and 10 are satisfied for the treatment of oral cancer, but there is less certainty regarding the management of OMPDs.

Oral Cancer and OPMDs: The Screening Program

There has been only one properly conducted randomized, controlled trial of a screening program for oral cancer that used mortality as the primary outcome. Sankaranarayanan et al. (36) conducted a fifteen-year, cluster-randomized controlled trial in the Trivandrum district of Kerala, India, to study the effect of visual screening (COE) on oral cancer mortality to assess whether this approach was sufficiently cost-effective for implementation in routine health care settings in high-risk populations such as those

Table 8.3. Advantages and Shortcomings of COE, and Possible Future Approaches

Advantages	Shortcomings	Future Approaches
• Is minimally invasive • Has high validity (sensitivity and specificity, in case of experienced examiners) • Is applicable in primary care setting • Requires minimum examination time once screener is trained • Can be repeated; has no morbidity • Requires no special facilities • Can be undertaken together with any other general and dental examinations	• May depend on the quality of the examiner • Requires training and calibration of screeners • Cannot distinguish among benign lesions, cancer, and OPMDs • May have low compliance, and screen positives may not present for secondary examinations • May not be cost-effective • Is difficult to maintain a simple record of	• Establish a clear definition of a positive screen and continuous training program • Develop scientifically evaluated, adjunctive tests or biomarkers • Develop basic strategies for health promotion, advocacy, enabling, and mediating. Need well-developed referral and monitoring. • Cost-effectiveness studies should be conducted • Photograph lesions; standardization may be desirable

in LMICS. The study population was categorized randomly into thirteen clusters: seven comprised the intervention group (n = 96,517) and six comprised the control group (n = 95,356). Healthy, asymptomatic subjects age thirty-five and older with no past history of oral cancer were included in the study. Intervention health workers (including university graduates in biology or social sciences) underwent three months of training to learn how to enumerate and identify eligible subjects; interview subjects to elicit socio-demographic factors, personal habits (such as chewing areca nut, smoking, and drinking alcohol), diet, and medical history; measure subjects' height, weight, blood pressure, and respiratory peak flow; and perform the COE on subjects in the intervention group. Subjects with clinical oral findings commensurate with oral cancer or OPMDs (those who were screen positive) were referred to a specialist. Subjects with confirmed oral cancers were referred for treatment with surgery, and/or radiotherapy, and/or chemotherapy. The

OPMDS underwent surgical excision wherever possible, and subjects with nonexcisable lesions were provided close follow-up treatment. Subjects with oral submucous fibrosis were treated symptomatically. Screen negative subjects were reexamined after three years. Control health workers were only responsible for enumeration, interviewing, and measurement of vital signs. They did not receive any training, nor did they perform COEs on the control subjects.

A detailed analysis of the outcomes was reported in 2005 after three rounds of screening (1996–2004). (37,38) The primary outcome was the difference in oral cancer mortality in the intervention and control groups. In the intervention arm, 91 percent were interviewed; 84 percent in the control arm were interviewed. Of the total, 87,655 individuals (91%) were screened at least once, and 5,145 (6.5%) screened positive. Of these, only 3,218 (62%) complied with referral. The detection rate of OPMDS or oral cancer was 28.0, 11.6, and 11.3 per 1,000 people screened in the first, second, and third rounds, respectively. In the intervention clusters, 205 cases of oral cancer were diagnosed (131 in screen-detected and referred, 59 interval cancers, and 15 in nonparticipants), and 158 cases were diagnosed in the control group. Seventy-seven people (37.6%) died of oral cancer in the intervention arm and eighty-seven people died (55%) in the control arm, but this difference was not statistically significant.

In the population as a whole there was no significant reduction in mortality (16.4% and 20.7%, respectively). However, there was a significant difference in five-year survival (intervention arm, 50%; control arm, 34%) and in the number of cases diagnosed in stages I and II (42% and 23%, respectively). The data were further analyzed to determine if the effects were greater in high-risk groups (defined as users of tobacco and/or alcohol). Among males who used tobacco and/or alcohol, there was a significant reduction in mortality, from 42.9 percent in the control group to 24.6 percent in the intervention group. There was no significant reduction among females in the study.

Results from a subsequent (fourth) round of screening completed in 2009 show that after four rounds there was a 12 percent reduction in overall mortality for the entire population, but this was not statistically significant. (39) However, the high-risk subjects (those with a history of tobacco and/or alcohol use) showed a significant, 21 percent reduction in mortality. Moreover, for all subjects who participated in all four cycles of screening (albeit only 20% of the eligible population), there was a significant reduction in mortality of 79 percent in the intervention group compared to the controls (17.1 per 100,000 reduced to 3.0). In high-risk subjects who underwent four rounds, the reduction in mortality was 81 percent (39 per 100,000 reduced to 7.1). In addition, there was an overall significant improvement in both the five- and ten-year survival rates and in early detection of oral cancer (a down-staging shift). The authors reported no severe adverse events as a consequence of screening, directing biopsies, or excision of lesions.

Subramanian et al. (40) looked at the costs of the Kerala trial. They estimated the total costs (in 2004 US dollars) for each group after three rounds of screening, as well as the incremental cost per life-year saved for all eligible individuals and for high-risk individuals (tobacco or alcohol users). Oral cancer screening by COE was performed for under US$6 per person. The total cost for the intervention category was US$478,742, compared to US$260,351 for the control group. The incremental cost per life-year saved was US$835 for all individuals eligible for screening and US$156 for high-risk individuals.

The data from the Kerala group demonstrate that oral cancer screening using COE, even in high-prevalence settings, did not reduce mortality in the population. The data do suggest, however, that screening of high-risk groups only (as opposed to the general population) in an LMIC such as India may be effective in reducing mortality. In terms of meeting criteria 11–14 (see table 8.2), these results suggest that oral cancer screening should not be recommended for the general population. Rather, there is value in screening high-risk individuals.

Oral Cancer and OPMDs: Implementation Criteria

To the best of our knowledge, only two countries currently operate formal oral cancer control programs: Cuba and Taiwan. The Cuban program was established in 1982 as part of a national oral cancer detection strategy. (41) This program is not a screening program in the strictest sense; rather, it is designated as a case finding, opportunistic program run in regional dental clinics across Cuba in which dentists perform COE on patients age fifteen or older (this age has subsequently been increased to age thirty-five or older). All "screen positive" patients with OPMDs are referred to an oral and maxillofacial surgeon for further evaluation, and all cancers are reported to the National Cancer Registry. Published results from the program during 1984–1990 demonstrated that a down-staging of oral cancers was equated with the implementation of the program. (42) However, similar to the results in the Kerala study, this program was not accompanied by a reduction in national oral cancer mortality rates. (43)

Taiwan's national oral cancer screening program, launched in 2004, was preceded by a series of oral cancer screening studies, the first phase of which was initiated in 1998–1999. More than 8,360 high-risk men who chewed areca nut were screened in twelve health units around Taipei City. There was a high prevalence of OPMDs in this population, with a dose-response relationship associated with the frequency of daily areca nut use. (44) Findings from this study led to the integration of screening for oral cancer and OPMDs into a community-based, multiple screening model designed and implemented in Keelung city, Taiwan (the Keelung Community-Based Integrated Screening [KCBIS] program). (45) In this study, conducted over a three-year period from 1999 to 2001, more than 10,500 adults were screened for oral cancer and OPMDs, yielding 2 oral cancers and 114 OMPDs. The Taiwanese national oral cancer screening program is subsidized by the government to screen adults age eighteen and older who have a tobacco-smoking or areca-nut-chewing habit. Implementation criteria 15–20 are impossible to meet given the paucity of organized, population-based oral cancer screening programs.

Thoughts Based on the Available Evidence

Based on the available evidence to date, the data seem to suggest that it is feasible to screen for oral cancer and OPMDs in LMICs. That being said, the conventional oral examination is the only oral cancer screening test that has been validated. This test is easy for even trained nonexperts to perform. It is painless and well accepted by patients; most important, it is inexpensive. However, while the COE demonstrates accuracy in detecting clinical lesions meeting the criteria for the clinical diagnosis of oral cancer or OPMDs, in reality the majority of "screen positive" lesions referred for evaluation by a specialist are not cancers per se, but OPMD lesions or disorders with uncertain malignant potential. Given the overall malignant transformation rate of < 5 percent, a "screen positive" COE is ultimately a poor surrogate marker for cancer or for lesions that have a significant likelihood for malignant transformation. Indeed, Speight et al. (46) conducted a value of information (VOI) analysis and concluded that the greatest source of uncertainty in determining the outcomes of oral cancer screening lay

Table 8.4. Suggested Priority Areas for Further Research

Natural history of the disease

Malignant transformation rates in OPMDs
Rates of progression through stages of disease from precancer to cancer
Clinical and molecular biomarkers of the high-risk lesion

Screening tests

Evaluation of adjunctive screening tests (e.g., salivary diagnostics)
Criteria for positive and negative tests
Evaluations in appropriate populations with sensitivity and specificity as endpoints
Evaluations of test accuracy among different groups of health workers

Screening programs

Further evaluations of programs: randomized clinical trials, but also simulation and
    demonstration studies
Evaluation of opportunistic screening programs in different settings
Identification of relevant high-risk groups and methods of targeting
Evaluation of risk reduction advice at time of screening

---

in our lack of understanding of malignant transformation of OPMD and disease progression.

Until there are advances in molecular screening or other screening adjuncts that can help narrow the pool of patients who are at the greatest risk for oral cancer, the COE remains the most viable screening test for LMICs. Creative solutions that allow stratification of "screen positive" patients into risk groups would allow resources to be strategically channeled to those patients with the highest risk. In an LMIC with a high prevalence of disease and limited resources (financial and provider) to diagnose and manage patients with oral cancer, adjunctive techniques that can accurately detect high-risk disease (such as early squamous cell carcinoma or high-grade dysplasia) would have the greatest clinical and economic utility. Point-of-care diagnostics seem more imperative in low-resource settings, where patient follow-up is challenging.

The use of telemedicine and mobile technology to facilitate the dissemination of information from the field is an attractive development, and we expect this area will evolve as the world becomes increasingly more connected. (47) Such ideas need to be empirically tested to assess their value. Table 8.4 presents some ideas that we offer for consideration. Because oral cancers are highly prevalent in many LMICs, and because these cancers generally have a poor prognosis, serious consideration should be given to implementing an oral cancer screening program targeting high-risk individuals so that suspicious lesions can be detected at an early, more treatable stage. Doing so would greatly improve the chances of survival. However, as is true of so many cancer screening programs, huge challenges must be overcome.

References

1. Sankaranarayanan R. Screening for cancer in low- and middle-income countries. Ann Glob Health 2014;80(5):412–7.

2. The World Bank. World development indicators map [cited 2016 Dec 20]. Available from: http://data.worldbank.org/products/wdi-maps.

3. United Kingdom Government. Guidance on criteria for appraising the viability, effectiveness and appropriateness of a screening programme. 2015 Oct 23 [cited 2016 Dec 20]. Available from: https://www.gov.uk/government/publications/evidence -review-criteria-national-screening-programmes/criteria-for-appraising-the -viability-effectiveness-and-appropriateness-of-a-screening-programme.

4. United States Preventive Services Task Force. Methods and processes [cited 2016 Dec 20]. Available from: https://www.uspreventiveservicestaskforce.org/Page/Name /methods-and-processes.

5. World Health Organization. Cancer country profiles 2014 [cited 2016 Dec 20]. Available from: http://www.who.int/cancer/country-profiles/en/.

6. Warnakulasuriya S, Johnson NW, van der Waal I. Nomenclature and classification of potentially malignant disorders of the oral mucosa. J Oral Pathol Med 2007;36(10):575–80.

7. Tilakaratne WM, Ekanayaka RP, Warnakulasuriya S. Oral submucous fibrosis: a historical perspective and a review on etiology and pathogenesis. Oral Surg Oral Med Oral Path Oral Radiol 2016; 122(2):178–91.

8. Ferlay J, Soerjomataram I, Dikshit R, et al. Cancer incidence and mortality worldwide: sources, methods and major patterns in GLOBOCAN 2012. Int J Cancer 2015;136(5):E359–86.

9. Seoane J, Alvarez-Novoa P, Gomez I, et al. Early oral cancer diagnosis: the Aarhus statement perspective; a systematic review and meta-analysis. Head Neck 2016;38(Suppl 1):E2182–9.

10. Napier SS, Speight PM. Natural history of potentially malignant oral lesions and conditions: an overview of the literature. J Oral Pathol Med 2008;37(1):1–10.

11. Petti S. Pooled estimate of world leukoplakia prevalence: a systematic review. Oral Oncol 2003;39(8):770–80.

12. Warnakulasuriya S, Ariyawardana A. Malignant transformation of oral leukoplakia: a systematic review of observational studies. J Oral Pathol Med 2016;45(3): 155–66.

13. Sankaranarayanan R, Ramadas K, Amarasinghe H, et al. Oral cancer: prevention, early detection, and treatment. In: Gelband H, Jha P, Sankaranarayanan R, Horton S, editors. Cancer: disease control priorities, Vol. 3. 3rd ed. Washington, DC: The International Bank for Reconstruction and Development/The World Bank; 2015. ch. 5.

14. Miles A, Cockburn J, Smith RA, Wardle J. A perspective from countries using organized screening programs. Cancer 2004;101(Suppl 5):1201–13.

15. AAOM clinical practice statement: subject: oral cancer examination and screening. Oral Surg Oral Med Oral Path Oral Radiol 2016;122(2):174–5.

16. Warnakulasuriya S. Lack of molecular markers to predict malignant potential of oral precancer. J Pathol 2000;190(4):407–9.

17. Rizzo G, Black M, Mymryk JS, et al. Defining the genomic landscape of head and neck cancers through next-generation sequencing. Oral Dis 2015;21(1):e11–24.

18. Wilson JMG, Jungner G. Principles and practice of screening for disease. Geneva: World Health Organization; 1968 [cited 2016 Dec 20]. Available from: http://apps.who.int/iris/bitstream/10665/37650/17/WHO_PHP_34.pdf.

19. Chang IH, Jiang RS, Wong YK, et al. Visual screening of oral cavity cancer in a male population: experience from a medical center. J Chin Med Assoc 2011;74(12): 561–6.

20. Warnakulasuriya S, Pindborg JJ. Reliability of oral precancer screening by primary health care workers in Sri Lanka. Commun Dent Health 1990;7(1):73–9.

21. Warnakulasuriya KA, Nanayakkara BG. Reproducibility of an oral cancer and precancer detection program using a primary health care model in Sri Lanka. Cancer Detect Prev 1991;15(5):331–4.

22. Mathew B, Sankaranarayanan R, Sunilkumar KB, et al. Reproducibility and validity of oral visual inspection by trained health workers in the detection of oral precancer and cancer. Brit J Cancer 1997;76(3):390–4.

23. Mehta FS, Gupta PC, Bhonsle RB, et al. Detection of oral cancer using basic health workers in an area of high oral cancer incidence in India. Cancer Detect Prev 1986;9(3–4):219–25.

24. Walsh T, Liu JL, Brocklehurst P, et al. Clinical assessment to screen for the detection of oral cavity cancer and potentially malignant disorders in apparently healthy adults. Cochrane Database Syst Rev 2013;(11):Cd010173.

25. Elango KJ, Anandkrishnan N, Suresh A, et al. Mouth self-examination to improve oral cancer awareness and early detection in a high-risk population. Oral Oncol 2011;47(7):620–4.

26. Scott SE, Rizvi K, Grunfeld EA, McGurk M. Pilot study to estimate the accuracy of mouth self-examination in an at-risk group. Head Neck 2010;32(10):1393–401.

27. Su WW, Yen AM, Chiu SY, Chen TH. A community-based RCT for oral cancer screening with toluidine blue. J Dent Res 2010;89(9):933–7.

28. Petti S. Oral cancer screening usefulness: between true and perceived effectiveness. Oral Dis 2016;22(2):104–8.

29. Singh V, Parashari A, Ahmed S, et al. Reasons for non-compliance of patients

to attend referral hospital after screening for oral pre-cancer lesions through camp approach in rural population of India. Ann Med Health Sci Res 2013;3(Suppl 1):S54–5.

30. Speight PM, Epstein J, Kujan O, et al. Screening for oral cancer—a perspective from the Global Oral Cancer Forum. Oral Surg Oral Med Oral Path Oral Radiol 2017;123(6):680–7. doi: 10.1016/j.0000.2016.08.021.

31. National Comprehensive Cancer Network. Clinical practice guidelines in oncology: head and neck cancers. 2016 [cited 2016 Dec 20]. Available from: https://www .nccn.org/professionals/physician_gls/PDF/head-and-neck.pdf.

32. D'Cruz A, Lin T, Anand AK, et al. Consensus recommendations for management of head and neck cancer in Asian countries: a review of international guidelines. Oral Oncol 2013;49(9):872–7.

33. Holmstrup P. Can we prevent malignancy by treating premalignant lesions? Oral Oncol 2009;45(7):549–50.

34. Lodi G, Franchini R, Warnakulasuriya S, et al. Interventions for treating oral leukoplakia to prevent oral cancer. Cochrane Database of Syst Rev 2016;7:Cd001829.

35. Mehanna HM, Rattay T, Smith J, McConkey CC. Treatment and follow-up of oral dysplasia—a systematic review and meta-analysis. Head Neck 2009;31(12): 1600–9.

36. Sankaranarayanan R, Mathew B, Jacob BJ, et al. Early findings from a community-based, cluster-randomized, controlled oral cancer screening trial in Kerala, India. The Trivandrum Oral Cancer Screening Study Group. Cancer 2000;88(3): 664–73.

37. Ramadas K, Sankaranarayanan R, Jacob BJ, et al. Interim results from a cluster randomized controlled oral cancer screening trial in Kerala, India. Oral Oncol 2003;39(6):580–8.

38. Sankaranarayanan R, Ramadas K, Thomas G, et al. Effect of screening on oral cancer mortality in Kerala, India: a cluster-randomised controlled trial. Lancet 2005;365(9475):1927–33.

39. Sankaranarayanan R, Ramadas K, Thara S, Muwonge R, Thomas G, Anju G, et al. Long-term effect of visual screening on oral cancer incidence and mortality in a randomized trial in Kerala, India. Oral Oncol 2013;49(4):314–21.

40. Subramanian IS, Sankaranarayanan IIR, Bapat IB, et al. Cost-effectiveness of oral cancer screening: results from a cluster randomized controlled trial in India. Bull World Health Organ 2009;87(3):200–6.

41. Gonzalez RS. Cancer screening: global debates and Cuban experience. MEDICC Rev 2014;16(3–4):73–7.

42. Santana JC, Delgado L, Miranda J, Sanchez M. Oral Cancer Case Finding Program (OCCFP). Oral Oncol 1997;33(1):10–2.

43. Fernandez Garrote L, Sankaranarayanan R, Lence Anta JJ, Rodriguez Salva A, Maxwell Parkin D. An evaluation of the oral cancer control program in Cuba. Epidemiol 1995;6(4):428–31.

44. Yen AM, Chen SC, Chen TH. Dose-response relationships of oral habits

associated with the risk of oral pre-malignant lesions among men who chew betel quid. Oral Oncol 2007;43(7):634–8.

45. Chen TH, Chiu YH, Luh DL, Yen MF, Wu HM, Chen LS, et al. Community-based multiple screening model: design, implementation, and analysis of 42,387 participants. Cancer 2004;100(8):1734–43.

46. Speight PM, Palmer S, Moles DR, Downer MC, Smith DH, Henriksson M, et al. The cost-effectiveness of screening for oral cancer in primary care. Health Technol Assess 2006;10(14):1–144, iii–iv.

47. Birur PN, Sunny SP, Jena S, Kandasarma U, Raghavan S, Ramaswamy B, et al. Mobile health application for remote oral cancer surveillance. J Am Dent Assoc 2015;146(12):886–94.

Chapter 9

Shreya Bhatt and Jay Evans

Mobile Health for Cancer Care and Control in Low- and Middle-Income Countries

Leveraging the Power of Mobile Technology
to Improve Cancer Outcomes

Introduction

Over the past few decades advances in global health and biomedical knowledge have made important contributions to saving lives. Yet 1 billion people living in last-mile and remote communities around the world still receive no medical care. (1) Many of the global health challenges we face today require solutions that improve and ensure the effective delivery and coordination of health care, particularly to these last-mile communities, where access to high-quality and affordable health care remains a pipe dream. However, a unique opportunity has emerged over the last decade that may help to address some of the challenges to the provision and coordination of care.

Mobile technology is the fastest growing technology in human history, reaching more people in developing countries than had been possible by other means of communication and connecting more people globally than even basic infrastructure such as road systems and power grids. In the short span of a decade, mobile cellular subscriptions have skyrocketed, with over 97 percent of the global population now living within reach of a mobile phone signal. (2) Penetrating the most remote corners of the world, the rapid expansion of mobile technology has created an unparalleled opportunity to extend basic health care services to remote and underserved populations, particularly in low- and middle-income countries (LMICs), where health care infrastructure and systems are often fragmented and ineffective. (3) Mobile technology for health, or mHealth, seeks to capitalize on this opportunity.

The mHealth Opportunity

In 2011 the World Health Organization (WHO) announced that mHealth has the potential to transform how health care is delivered around the world. (4) While there is no established and standardized definition of mHealth, (5) it broadly refers to the use of wireless information and communication devices (such as mobile phones and personal digital assistants [PDAs]) and mobile phone networks for medical and public health practice. Depending on the prevailing context and infrastructure, mHealth interventions harness core functionalities of mobile phones, such as voice and short messaging service (SMS), as well as more complex functionalities and applications, such as third- and fourth-generation mobile telecommunication systems, global positioning systems, and Bluetooth technology.

Since its inception mHealth technology has grown rapidly, and new mHealth interventions have proliferated, with over 500 pilot programs deployed globally, many of which are concentrated in Asia and sub-Saharan Africa. (6) mHealth interventions are designed to address health care challenges faced by patients, communities, and practitioners, including access, quality, and affordability, and serve to not only strengthen health systems but also improve health outcomes. (7) Because of the heterogeneity in health care challenges, mHealth interventions are by design dynamic and often vary in their applications, outcomes, and impact. (8)

One of the most common uses of mHealth is to facilitate *communication* among patients, health workers, and facility-based care providers, particularly when access to treatment is limited, costly, or difficult, as is the case in many LMICs. In these settings, mobile technology has been used to change behaviors and attitudes by improving treatment compliance (9,10) and promoting the use of health services and encouraging preventive behavior. (11,12)

Data collection and reporting is another common application of mHealth in low-resource settings. Such interventions allow frontline workers to collect data in real time using technology rather than traditional paper-based systems, to improve operational efficiencies by saving hours of their time and lowering costs, (13) and to perform real-time supervision of performance and quality control. (14) The use of mHealth for real-time data collection has also been crucial in monitoring disease outbreaks, emergencies, and disaster management situations; mobile technologies have overcome communication and accessibility barriers to track incidents, offer information on available services, and help responders target resources more effectively. (15)

Another common use of mHealth is *care coordination*. Mobile tools can be used to support frontline workers and care providers in tracking vital events, delivering timely care, prioritizing services, and ensuring effective case management over time. A range of mHealth interventions for maternal and child health, for example, allows frontline workers to register pregnancies and births using mobile tools and track antenatal care appointments, deliveries, birth outcomes, vaccination appointments, nutrition, and followups more effectively, improving maternal and neonatal health outcomes. (16,17)

mHealth interventions have also been used for a variety of other purposes that may not directly engage with patients but aim to improve access to and quality of care. These applications include the use of mHealth interventions for continuing medical training and education for frontline and remote care providers; point-of-care decision support tools for frontline workers; supply chain management of essential medication and medical equipment for remote clinics; electronic health records to maintain longitudinal patient histories; and human resource or performance management of community health workers, who often have intermittent access to supervisory staff. (18)

At its core, each of these applications of mHealth interventions, be it for communication, data collection, care coordination, decision support, or performance management, has the same overarching objectives: to address the health care challenges of access, quality, and affordability for the many disconnected and underserved populations in low-resource settings, to provide support for health systems, and to improve health outcomes. What role, then, can mHealth play when it comes to improving cancer outcomes around the world?

mHealth and Cancer Care

Since its inception, mHealth interventions implemented in LMICs have focused on improving health outcomes in areas such as maternal and child health and infectious diseases. However, there are very few evidence-based mHealth interventions implemented for non-communicable diseases (NCDs) in low-resource settings. (19) These diseases pose one of the greatest health challenges of the twenty-first century, primarily due to a confluence of forces, including an aging population and changes in lifestyle and diet. (20) Cancer, in particular, disproportionately affects people in LMICs, where more than 60 percent of all global cancer deaths occur. (21) In most LMICs, the health care system is particularly weak and ill-equipped to meet this growing burden. (22)

Health care infrastructure for cancer care and control in LMICs is often fragmented. There is little primary prevention, screening, and treatment, and there is an acute shortage of qualified health professionals skilled in cancer detection and diagnosis. Treatment is limited or nonexistent. Compounding matters, LMICs tend to have poor referral systems among primary, secondary, and tertiary care facilities. (23,24) Moreover, low-resource communities face many barriers to treatment, including financial constraints; prohibitive distances from health facilities; and sociocultural barriers such as lack of awareness, a fear of cancer, and poor health literacy, in which cancer is associated with many myths and stigma, and with death. Unfortunately many patients living in LMICs will seek care at health care facilities at late stages of their cancer, often when the condition is no longer curable. (25,26) They often face lengthy, complex, and costly journeys to seek care, assuming that they seek care at all. Experience has shown that even in such challenging settings, cancer care is possible with the use of innovative mHealth solutions that improve care coordination, enhance access to care, and strengthen health systems to meet the growing burden of cancer.

A Case Study: Low-cost Mobile Technology for Cervical and Oral Cancer Screening in Rural India

In 2015 Medic Mobile, a nonprofit technology organization that builds mobile tools to improve health care delivery in low-resource settings, began a partnership with the University of Edinburgh, Weill Cornell Medical College, and Christian Medical College, Vellore, to pilot an mHealth intervention for cervical and oral cancer screening in rural India. Like many developing countries, India faces a severe shortage of skilled health professionals in rural areas. There are only seven doctors for every 10,000 citizens, and these professionals are heavily concentrated in urban centers, even though two-thirds of the country's population lives in rural settings. (27) India, like many LMICs, is dealing with the dual burden of communicable diseases and a growing burden of NCDs, especially cancer, cardiovascular disease, and diabetes. It is probably an understatement to say that delivering cancer care through prevention, screening, diagnosis, treatment, and palliative support services to underserved and remote rural populations is a major challenge.

Cervical and oral cancer constitute the two most common cancers in India for women and men, respectively, despite the fact that both cancers are amenable to treatment; cervical cancer accounts for nearly 26 percent of all new cancer cases diagnosed in India. (28) The incidence of oral cancer is the highest of any cancer among Indian men. (29) Low-resource communities in India face the same challenges in access to care as do other LMICs, including economic, logistical, social, and cultural barriers that significantly delay care-seeking behavior and result in late-stage presentation at primary care centers. (30)

As part of a pilot study, Medic Mobile designed and implemented an mHealth prototype to strengthen community-based cervical and oral cancer screening and follow-up services at three rural mission hospitals in the states of Tamil Nadu, Madhya Pradesh, and Chhattisgarh. These hospitals provide care to extremely underserved and low-income populations and are the only hospitals in their vicinities. Given financial constraints, a lack of awareness, limited understanding of the gravity of the disease, fear, and social inhibition on the part of patients and communities, these hospitals often bear witness to late-stage presentation of cancer and other potentially treatable conditions. (31)

The pilot study aimed to explore how low-cost mHealth solutions could support care coordination in such resource-poor settings. A group of twenty health workers, nurses, and coordinators across the three sites were equipped with low-cost mobile phones. They were trained in how to use these devices, to report on the results of cervical and oral cancer screenings they conducted, and to report on subsequent interactions with patients, including facility visits for a biopsy and treatment.

Since the launch of the pilot program in 2015, health workers and nurses have relied on inexpensive, basic phones that are ubiquitous and functional even in areas with limited infrastructure and connectivity. By using simple technology such as text messaging and menu-driven applications on these phones, health workers and nurses can keep track of participants in the screening program more effectively than by using traditional paper-based methods. Within the first six months of the pilot, more than 1,700 cervical and oral cancer screenings were conducted using the mHealth tools in 130 villages. Of these, 220 screening results were positive. Initial qualitative feedback from the community health workers and nurses is very promising. Health workers and nurses found that whereas maintaining traditional paper-based records was time-consuming and tedious, using mobile phones for such reporting was quick and easy and enhanced their efficiency, which benefited not only the health workers but also the communities they serve. Feedback from program coordinators was equally positive. The mHealth intervention allowed them to get an accurate, real-time picture of the screening activities and data. The program enabled the workers to follow up in a timely fashion with positive cases who had not yet sought treatment at the facilities.

This intervention illustrates how mHealth solutions can improve health worker efficiency and care coordination and support providers in extending cancer care to disconnected communities in low-resource settings. It also illustrates that mHealth interventions need not always leverage the latest and most expensive mobile technology available, such as tablets or smartphones. Simple, low-cost, low-technology tools such as basic phones and text messaging can serve a useful purpose in resource-constrained settings.

Opportunities for mHealth in the Cancer Care Continuum: How Mobile Tools Can Be Used to Improve Quality of Cancer Care in LMICS

Health systems in LMICS require coordination among various levels of care, including community-based care at the village or community level, health center– or clinic-based care at the primary level, hospitals at the secondary level, and referral centers or larger hospitals at the tertiary level. (32) (See figure 9.1.) Experience shows that mHealth tools can strengthen care coordination at various points throughout the cancer care continuum, including prevention, screening, early diagnosis, treatment, and palliative care, and across the various levels of health care systems in LMICS.

Prevention

mHealth interventions for cancer prevention, particularly in the form of behavioral-change communication for smoking cessation, have been shown to be effective in high-income countries such as New Zealand and Norway. (33) Similar interventions can be applied in LMICS to create positive

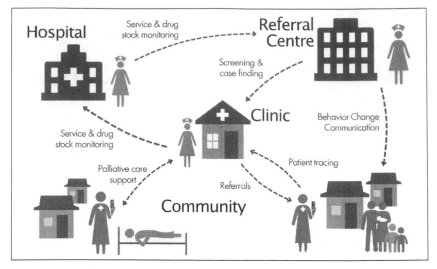

Figure 9.1. Care coordination across multiple levels of health systems in LMICs and the opportunities for mHealth in the cancer care continuum

behavioral changes by reinforcing the cessation of smoking and other risk factors and by encouraging preventative behaviors such as HPV vaccinations in settings where these services are available. (34) Behavioral change communication interventions are often text message or SMS based. Estimates suggest that 98 percent of all cell phones worldwide have SMS capabilities, making text messages available on nearly every model of mobile phone, whether old or new, including the basic phones that are predominantly used in many remote areas in LMICs. (35) Moreover, text messages are usually inexpensive, require minimal bandwidth, and do not require significant technological expertise to view on the part of the recipient. Information sent through text messages can be received at any time, even if the mobile phone is temporarily turned off, and can be accessed repeatedly, as and when the recipient chooses.

While text messages hold strong promise for communicating key behavioral change messages, they require careful consideration with regard to the audience's preferences in language, timing, health needs, and confidentiality, as well as sociocultural norms of behavior and messaging in the audience's context. (36) This is especially important with regard to female cancers. There are 200 million fewer female mobile phone subscribers than male subscribers in LMICs, and the gender gap is more pronounced in parts of the world such as South Asia, where women are 38 percent less likely to own a phone than are men. (37) In such settings, communicating sensitive behavioral change information related to female cancers, such as promoting HPV vaccinations or preventing risk factors of cervical cancer, via text messages may violate the audience's need for privacy and confidentiality, especially when women only have partial access to phones that are often controlled by male members of their families. Despite these limitations, we believe that text messages offer an opportunity to communicate culturally appropriate and context-relevant behavioral change information and reinforcement. Further research is needed to test the efficacy of such messages for cancer prevention in LMICs.

Screening and Early Diagnosis

Several mHealth pilots have involved community-based screening for communicable and chronic diseases in LMICs. For example, in a pilot program at St. Gabriel's Hospital in Malawi, community health workers used text messages to communicate with nurses at the hospital and were able to screen, detect, and refer twice as many tuberculosis patients as before the pilot. (38) In another mHealth pilot program in South Africa, community health workers using a feature phone tool were able to screen for cardiovascular diseases 40 percent faster than when using conventional paper-based screening methods, and perhaps more striking, the training time for the use of these mobile tools was 76 percent shorter than it was for the paper-based screening tool. (39) In a pilot program focused on oral cancer in India, rural health workers used a smartphone-based application to screen for precancerous and cancerous lesions and to transmit medical data in the form of text, audio, video, or photos to a remote medical specialist for real-time decision support. (40)

These examples highlight that a range of mobile devices and technologies, from basic-feature phones and text messaging to more complex smartphone-based applications, can be efficiently and easily used by health workers and primary care providers for screening and detection of a variety of conditions, including cancer care. Simple feature phone applications can record patient information and relevant behaviors such as smoking or drinking habits, creating digital patient screening records that can be easily and quickly communicated to facility-based staff. Smartphone applications, on the other hand, may employ more complex decision support programming to guide health workers in early diagnosis. Such applications may use algorithms based on predetermined care protocols to analyze reported symptoms or visual content such as images of lesions and provide health workers with decision support on appropriate next steps for that interaction, such as referrals to the facility. This immediate decision support at the time of screening reduces the number of patient revisits to the facility, as health workers are able to inform patients of screening results and diagnose in real time. Moreover, compared to paper-based systems of screening, mHealth technology can save significant time that would otherwise be spent on personnel training, record keeping, and administration. Thus, health workers can be available to screen more people more efficiently in a shorter period of time.

Treatment and Management of Patient Care Pathways

mHealth solutions can also facilitate and manage care pathways once patients enter the treatment cycle. Various mHealth pilot programs in high-income settings have used automated text messages to remind patients of upcoming appointments in a bid to improve clinic attendance and reduce dropout rates. (41,42) Patient adherence to treatment recommendations has significantly improved. A randomized control trial in Kenya showed that HIV/AIDS patients receiving SMS reminders promoting adherence to antiretroviral therapy had significantly improved adherence rates and rates of viral suppression compared to the control group. (43) In a similar mHealth study promoting adherence to antiretroviral therapy among a cohort of HIV/AIDS patients in India, not only did the messaging improve adherence, but the improvement was also found to have a lasting effect for at least six months after the intervention ended. (44)

Similar interventions that employ SMS or voice calls to send treatment reminders can also be implemented for cancer care in LMICs. Traditional approaches to cancer care, such as conventional screening and treatment, often require three or more visits to a health center, which poses challenges for low-resource communities, resulting in dropouts and poor health outcomes. (45) Using mHealth tools to send reminders for upcoming or missed appointments for biopsy tests and results, treatment visits, and other follow-up appointments can reduce dropouts and loss to follow-up between key points of the patient-provider interaction. Moreover, these messages and calls can be tailored according to the context and can be sent directly to patients and family caregivers, to community health workers who can reinforce the reminders with the patients in person, or to both.

Service and Drug Stock Monitoring

mHealth interventions have been shown to have significant impact on the monitoring of care services provided by health workers and the supply of essential medication and medical equipment, particularly at rural health facilities, strengthening the supply chain and improving access to and quality of care in last-mile settings. The sMs for Life project in rural Tanzania, for example, used text messages and electronic mapping technology to facilitate accurate and comprehensive stock counts of antimalarial drugs at 129 rural health facilities on a weekly basis. This system reduced instances when the drugs were out of stock from 78 percent in the first week of the pilot to 26 percent in the last week. (46) Similar mHealth pilots for stock monitoring of antimalarial drugs have been implemented in Kenya (47) and Uganda, (48) both of which have showed improvements in the availability of life-saving drugs at rural facilities with the use of basic mobile phones. Such interventions can be applied in the realm of cancer care to report on stock levels of key cancer medication, particularly pain medication for palliative care patients, ensuring that the drugs are readily available at rural health posts so that patients can receive their medication when they need it.

mHealth interventions have also been used to monitor and enhance performance levels of care providers such as community health workers. A pilot program in Kenya found that sending text message reminders to community health workers improved and maintained their adherence to treatment guidelines for pediatric malaria by 23 percent. (49) A separate program in Tanzania using sMs reminders to improve the promptness of community health workers' home visits found that the reminders led to an 86 percent reduction in the average number of days that a health worker visit was overdue. (50) In the context of cancer care, similar interventions can be applied to enhance health worker performance in terms of conducting screenings and follow-up patient visits and to introduce greater accountability and transparency into health systems in low-resource settings.

Palliative Care

mHealth interventions can play an important role in facilitating palliative care and pain management to minimize patient suffering in cases where cancer treatment is unfeasible. A study of three palliative care programs in Uganda, Kenya, and Malawi in which mobile phones were used to strengthen linkages among nurses, health workers, patients, and their family caregivers found that access to competent palliative care was greatly expanded due to the use of mHealth. (51) mHealth interventions that facilitate two-way communication, such as voice calls, SMS, and instant messaging, and group messaging are often more appropriate in a palliative care context, as two-way dialogue helps to create an ongoing line of communication and enables patients to feel secure in their care environment.

These and several other ongoing demonstration projects suggest that mobile tools such as feature phones, smartphones, and tablets can use simple and inexpensive communication methods, including SMS and voice calls, as well as other more complex and costly software applications, to improve care coordination for cancer care and control in low-resource settings of LMICs. In light of the limited evidence on impact, however, there is a pressing need to build on the current research and apply learnings from mHealth in other health areas to cancer care in LMICs.

Designing mHealth Solutions for the Last Mile: A Human-Centered Design Approach

mHealth interventions are not only complex but can often look and feel significantly different from one context to the next. They also continuously evolve over the course of an implementation because technology changes rapidly, as do the needs of stakeholders. A successful mHealth intervention for HIV or tuberculosis drug adherence in Kenya may not necessarily prove equally effective for cancer control in India. Adapting mHealth interventions from one health area or context to another calls for the application of intelligent and adaptive design thinking principles that can take into account differing sociocultural contexts and care systems.

Design thinking is an approach to creating human-centered, systemic solutions for complex and systemic challenges. (52) It draws on a variety of fields, such as design studies, engineering, and human-computer interaction, as well as participatory design and the social sciences. (53) While there is no single blueprint for human-centered design, (54) these principles reflect an overall approach toward technology and innovation that puts people first. Design thinking places an emphasis on understanding the needs of the *people* who will use that system (also known as the *users*) as well as the context in which the system will be delivered. This allows for a ground-up approach to design, rather than one based on preconceptions or rigid rules of developers and system builders. (55)

Iterative and experimental in nature, the design thinking process typically involves three key and often overlapping stages: inspiration, ideation, and implementation. (56,57) *Inspiration* refers to the stage of immersion by observing, listening to, and spending time with people who will use the intervention, in order to foster a better understanding of their ecosystem, hopes, desires, and challenges and inspire the search for solutions that address those challenges. (58) In the course of this stage, one might discover that a female community health worker enjoys interacting with people, owns a basic phone, and is comfortable with the use of mobile technology, or perhaps that a nurse at a primary care center is often tired due to an overwhelmingly busy work schedule. Through these discoveries, the designer creates a *user persona*, or a character that embodies a particular type of user, such as a community health worker, enabling the designer to ground future ideation and implementation in the needs, priorities, motivations, and values of the users.

Ideation can be thought of as the stage of engaging with users to create and test ideas or prototypes to see what works and what does not and to uncover unexpected barriers as well as opportunities. In this stage, the user observations and stories collected during the inspiration stage are mined and analyzed to identify opportunities for design. As the name suggests, this stage leads to the generation of many ideas, some of which may be useful and practical, while others may be less feasible and are discarded as the design process continues. Initial prototypes of promising ideas are created to share with users for their feedback and are refined and iterated until a final solution emerges that meets the needs of the users and addresses the gaps and/or challenges they face. (59) For example, ideas to improve prevention of cancer in a low-resource community may include behavioral change communications on smoking cessation sent directly to community members. In settings where mobile phone ownership is low, however, the solution that creates a deeper impact may be one that is targeted to the village elders and health workers, who will then reinforce the messaging in person.

In the final stage of *implementation*, the "best ideas" generated during ideation are shaped into actual products and services and are introduced to the users to effect positive change. Partnerships are forged with key stakeholders, including community leaders, self-help groups, and other collectives, to ensure support. Training and capacity building are conducted for the various users groups. In the context of cancer care, this may include community health workers, nurses and other facility-based staff, and program coordinators and supervisors. Finally, the intervention is launched and a strong monitoring and evaluation plan is put in place to measure the efficacy of the intervention over the course of its life.

Every stage of this often chaotic and multilayered journey requires the active participation of stakeholders to improve existing systems or to develop new ones that address unmet needs. However, it is not user consideration or participation alone that makes an approach to designing technology human-centered. The term can also imply a more conceptual commitment to enhance the skills and expertise of people within a system by using technology in a way that empowers them. (60) It can also stand for value-sensitive design, which emphasizes that user perspectives have an intrinsic value that is desirable in and of itself regardless of the other goals of implementing technology. (61)

The notion that user perspectives in developing and implementing interventions are valuable is not unique to mHealth. In a review of community engagement in cancer control studies among indigenous people of Australia, New Zealand, Canada, and the United States, researchers found that genuinely involving beneficiaries through all stages of an intervention led to a range of positive outcomes that included increased community capacity and empowerment, improved screening participation rates, and greater awareness of cancer-related services. (62) Involving community stakeholders in program development and implementation is also recognized as a strategy to increase and sustain the demand for services such as screenings and improve the quality of care, which in turn can result in greater screening participation and treatment compliance. (63) It would not be unreasonable to expect similar positive outcomes of engaging users during the design and implementation of mHealth interventions for cancer care.

Human-centered research and development for mHealth interventions have long been practiced in high-income countries. (64) As digital technologies continue to evolve and spread extensively in LMICs, the need for rigorous evaluation has become increasingly important. A movement spearheaded by several eminent global institutions, including United Nations agencies and the World Bank, has led to the creation and endorsement of nine principles guiding digital development, in which the first principle emphasizes the importance of designing with the user. (65) With the growing recognition of the importance of human-centered design for mHealth, it is time for the global health community to explore how these guiding principles might be used to adapt mHealth for cancer care and control in last-mile settings around the world, potentially saving the lives of many who suffer from or who are at risk for cancer.

mHealth Enablers: What Makes mHealth Interventions Successful?

Despite the strong promise that well-designed mHealth tools can improve health outcomes, the narrative around mHealth has become increasingly tempered by an air of cautious optimism. Even after the completion of over 500 pilot studies, little is known about the likely uptake, efficacy, and effectiveness of mHealth interventions. (66,67) Evidence from several contexts reveals that mHealth pilots have not fared well in terms of evolving into the well-established, sustainable, and impactful programs envisioned. In Uganda, twenty-three of thirty-six mHealth initiatives, or nearly 64 percent of the interventions in 2008 and 2009, failed to scale after the pilot phase. In India, more than thirty mHealth initiatives in 2009 were unsuccessful in progressing beyond the pilot stage. (68)

Empirical data suggest that mHealth pilot programs fail to scale due to a range of systemic faults, including flawed business and partnership models and funding schemes, as well as the lack of rigorous monitoring and evaluation to assess the effectiveness of these interventions. (69,70) While this highlights systemic gaps, there is a need for a closer look at what really makes mHealth interventions successful. What are the key *enablers* that create a conducive environment in which mHealth pilots can succeed, flourish, and grow into sustainable and impactful programs?

mHealth interventions are often regarded as complex endeavors, because they engage a wide variety of people, processes, and systems to improve health outcomes and because their success depends on changes in human behavior and in systems of care. (71) In our experience of designing and deploying over sixty mHealth interventions in more than twenty countries, we have found that several elements play a key role in making mHealth a success. These can be broadly categorized as the "Four Ps": people, pathways, platforms, and partnerships.

People

Perhaps one of the most important enablers of mHealth success is the human resources that support these interventions, and chief among these is a mHealth champion or leader (either an individual or a group of individuals who persistently drive the initiative forward). (72) As all complex systems do, mHealth interventions require effective management and supervision to ensure their success, particularly when there is still a lack of understanding about what types of mHealth interventions work, how, why, and in what conditions and contexts. (73)

In the effort to bring technology, people, and processes together, mHealth initiatives often encounter roadblocks such as changes in infrastructure or local context, unanticipated difficulties in human behavioral change, and unexpected technological issues. In such cases, a champion can serve as a crucial resource to address real-time implementation challenges, supervise frontline workers, and track the impact of the tools throughout the life of an intervention, with a view to course-correcting as needed and ensuring that the intervention achieves its stated goals.

A typical mHealth champion is an individual who plays a management or supervisory role within an implementing organization (such as a community health worker supervisor or program manager). Often working from health facilities or offices, the champion's role is to support frontline workers and facility-based staff in delivering health programs to underserved populations. While these champions may not have clinical experience or direct contact with the communities they serve, their managerial and problem-solving expertise is highly valued. Perhaps most important, however, they possess a strong will and commitment to making an mHealth intervention a success despite the many unanticipated challenges and barriers faced during an implementation. The champions also view the mobile intervention as serving to improve health outcomes, not just as a data collection or management tool. This shift in vision allows them to take into consideration user needs, which are also at the core of successfully scaled mHealth interventions. (74) The mHealth champion user persona, therefore, is one of the most important enablers of mHealth success.

Equally important to ensuring the success of mHealth interventions is a well-trained and skilled workforce with the capacity to support the implementation, use, and maintenance of mHealth tools. (75,76) This implies the need for a concerted effort to educate health care professionals, including frontline workers and facility-based staff such as nurses and doctors, about the potential role that mHealth technology can play in improving health care. (77) As more mHealth interventions are implemented each year, there is an urgent need for mHealth training programs for health personnel at all levels to ensure sustainability.

Pathways

While human resources play an undeniably important role in the success of mHealth interventions, an important enabler, and to a large extent a prerequisite for success particularly in the context of mHealth for cancer care and control, is the presence of well-defined and stable pathways to care. mHealth interventions are often viewed as a means to strengthen existing health systems to improve health outcomes. (78) However, if these systems are underdeveloped or inconsistent to begin with, simply layering technology onto these systems cannot have any meaningful impact and often can amplify existing systemic flaws. (79)

Pathways to cancer care and control in low-resource settings around the world are often fragmented. Remote populations in these settings have limited access to screening, diagnostic and treatment facilities, and cancer drugs and pain medication. Referral systems between disconnected segments of the cancer care pathway are often weak and ineffective. (80) When technology is introduced into such fragmented systems of care in low-resource settings, there may be a potential for the interventions not only to fail, but also to do more harm than good. An mHealth intervention for cervical cancer screening, for example, can help to identify precancerous lesions at an early stage so that patients have a better chance of receiving timely treatment and ultimately improved chances of survival. But if patients lack clear pathways to care (including access to affordable, life-saving treatments such as surgery, radiotherapy, or chemotherapy), the intervention will probably fail to improve health outcomes. (81)

It is important to note that technology alone often is not sufficient. Introducing an mHealth intervention in a cervical cancer screening program will not result in a greater number of women being screened and referred for treatment without context-relevant education and sensitive awareness-building campaigns that educate the population about the benefits of the program. While mHealth continues to hold strong promise for improving health outcomes in resource-poor settings, it cannot be viewed as a silver bullet or panacea for all the problems of poorly functioning health systems in these contexts. (82,83) Processes and pathways to care must be stable and well-defined for any technology intervention to succeed.

Platforms

In addition to skilled human resources and stable processes, the nature of the platform in mHealth interventions can determine success, particularly in terms of the opportunity to scale from small pilots to sustainable programs. While many mHealth interventions appear simple, their success and ability to reach a wider audience depend on how well such initiatives can communicate and integrate with other existing systems of care. (84)

Traditional approaches to information technology and health information systems are based on the use of devices that cannot communicate with one another, creating siloed and stand-alone technology solutions. (85) Such an approach may not reflect the typical patient experience and journey within the continuum of care, as patients often have multiple clinical needs and conditions at one time and interact with multiple points within a health system, including private and public providers. (86) Unlike stand-alone and bespoke solutions, enabling platforms can be thought of as systems that allow for the exchange of data between systems, use common protocols, and can work together. They integrate into existing health systems, leverage synergies, address communication gaps, and complement those systems' ultimate goals of delivering quality care through an efficient health workforce and improving health outcomes. (87) Interoperable platforms that can support and strengthen existing health systems rather than create parallel and detached solutions have a much greater chance of achieving larger-scale effectiveness and success in improving health outcomes.

Partnerships

Complex programs require effective coordination and partnership between key stakeholders if they are to succeed. mHealth interventions are no different. Any given mHealth intervention involves several partners, including mHealth providers, private health care providers, government care systems, mobile network operators, and donors. With the wide range of actors involved, many well-meaning mHealth interventions often face challenges due to ineffective cooperation among partners or differing goals and visions among them. While mobile network operators seek to maximize profits, government interests lie in improved health outcomes, and for-profit mHealth and/or technology providers seek to advance their respective technology products. Financing is a particularly striking challenge for many mHealth interventions, as pilot programs or proof of concept projects are often loss-making or supported by short- or medium-term grants, with limited long-term private and public funding channels to support these initiatives going forward. (88) As a result, sustainability is often a challenge for mHealth interventions. It would be helpful if governments, industry, and donors worked collaboratively to set industry standards and create a conducive environment in which mHealth programs can thrive. (89,90) The success of mHealth interventions depends on strong alliances among partners and the availability of sustainable funding mechanisms over the long term.

Conclusion: mHealth Priorities for the Future

Over the last decade mHealth technology has done much to help change the way health care is delivered in low-resource settings globally. Mobile phones have the potential to increase access, enhance quality, and improve patient adherence and compliance. They also can facilitate communication, data collection, care coordination, and decision support, as well as enhance health worker performance and improve medical supply chains.

As the increase in cancer incidence continues to overburden LMICs, it is increasingly important to adopt a multipronged mHealth agenda that can serve to strengthen health systems in these countries. First, there is a need for greater implementation of well-designed mHealth interventions to strengthen the prevention, screening, early diagnosis, and treatment of cancer in low-resource settings. mHealth pilot programs implemented in other health areas and contexts offer vast experiential learning, which must be adapted for cancer by using human-centered design principles. (91) Second, governments, donors, and other institutional actors need to set standards for common mHealth evaluation methodologies and metrics, and researchers and practitioners must place a greater emphasis on scientific evaluation of mHealth interventions to pave the way for future adoption at scale. Finally, institutional partners should work together to establish a global mHealth network that would enable the sharing of information on interventions, tools, and best practices; forge partnerships; and create an ecosystem in which mHealth can evolve in a more coordinated manner. (92)

Low-resource communities in LMICs face complex journeys to cancer care. Improving outcomes in these communities does not require medical innovations or the discovery of new drugs, but rather stronger care coordination and innovative methods of health care delivery. Mobile technology in the form of simple, low-cost tools and more advanced applications offers an opportunity to fill the communication and coordination gaps and enhance health care delivery in these settings. With a clear and progressive mHealth agenda and support from government, industry, and other interested partners, mobile technology can strengthen LMIC health systems and equip them to address the burden of disease, particularly among those living in remote, poor areas of the world.

References

1. World Health Organization. The global push for universal health coverage. 2014 [cited 2016 Nov 15]. Available from: http://www.who.int/health_financing/Global PushforUHC_final_11Jul14-1.pdf.

2. International Telecommunications Union. ICT facts & figures: the world in 2015. 2015 [cited 2016 Nov 15]. Available from: https://www.itu.int/en/ITU-D/Statistics /Documents/facts/ICTFactsFigures2015.pdf.

3. Mills A. Health care systems in low-and middle-income countries. N Engl J Med 2014;370(6):552–7.

4. Kay M, Santos J, Takane M. mHealth: new horizons for health through mobile technologies. World Health Organization 2011;64(7):66–71.

5. Ibid.

6. Boston Consulting Group and Telenor Group. Socio-economic impact of mHealth. 2012 Apr [cited 2016 Nov 15]. Available from: http://www.telenor.com /wp-content/uploads/2012/05/BCG-Telenor-Mobile-Health-Report-May-20121.pdf.

7. Labrique A B, Vasudevan L, Kochi E, et al. mHealth innovations as health system strengthening tools: 12 common applications and a visual framework. Glob Health Sci Pract 2013;1(2):160–71.

8. Phillips G, Felix L, Galli L, et al. The effectiveness of M-health technologies for improving health and health services: a systematic review protocol. BMC Res Notes 2010;Oct 6;3:250. doi: 10.1186/1756-0500-3-250.

9. Lester RT, Ritvo P, Mills EJ, et al. Effects of a mobile phone short message service on antiretroviral treatment adherence in Kenya (WelTel Kenya 1): a randomised trial. Lancet 2010;376(9755):1838–45.

10. Haberer JE, Robbins G K, Ybarra M, et al. Real-time electronic adherence monitoring is feasible, comparable to unannounced pill counts, and acceptable. AIDS Behav 2012;16(2):375–82.

11. Leach-Lemens, C. Using mobile phones in HIV care and prevention. HIV/AIDS Treat Pract 2009;137:7.

12. Vodopivec Jamsek V, de Jongh T, Gurol Urganci I, et al. Mobile phone messaging for preventive health care. Cochrane Database Syst Rev 2012;Dec 12;12:CD007457. doi: 10.1002/14651858.CD007457.pub2.

13. Mahmud N, Rodriguez J, Nesbit J. A text message-based intervention to bridge the healthcare communication gap in the rural developing world. Technol Health Care 2010;18(2):137–44.

14. Tomlinson M, Solomon W, Singh Y, et al. The use of mobile phones as a data collection tool: a report from a household survey in South Africa. BMC Med Inform Decis Mak 2009;Dec 23;9:51. doi: 10.1186/1472–6947-9-51.

15. Heinzelman J., Waters C. Crowdsourcing crisis information in disaster-affected Haiti. US Institute of Peace; 2010 [cited 2016 Nov 15]. Available from: http://www.usip.org/publications/crowdsourcing-crisis-information-in-disaster-affected-haiti.

16. Philbrick WC. mHealth and MNCH: state of the evidence—trends, gaps, stakeholder needs, and opportunities for future research on the use of mobile technology to improve maternal, newborn, and child health. mHealth Alliance, UN Foundation; 2013.

17. Rotheram-Borus MJ, Le Roux IM, Tomlinson M, et al. Philani Plus (+): a mentor mother community health worker home visiting program to improve maternal and infants' outcomes. Prev Sci 2011;12(4):372–88.

18. Labrique, Vasudevan, Kochi, et al., op. cit.

19. Holeman I, Evans J, Kane D, et al. Mobile health for cancer in low to middle income countries: priorities for research and development. Eur J Cancer Care 2014; 23(6):750–6.

20. World Health Organization. Global status report on noncommunicable diseases. 2014 [cited 2016 Sep 12]. Available from: http://www.who.int/nmh/publications/ncd-status-report-2014/en/.

21. International Agency for Research on Cancer. GLOBOCAN 2012: estimated cancer incidence, mortality and prevalence worldwide in 2012 [cited 2016 Sep 12]. Available from: http://globocan.iarc.fr/Pages/fact_sheets_cancer.aspx.

22. Farmer P, Frenk J, Knaul FM, et al. Expansion of cancer care and control in countries of low and middle income: a call to action. Lancet 2010;376(9747):1186–93.

23. CanTreat, International. Scaling up cancer diagnosis and treatment in developing countries: what can we learn from the HIV/AIDS epidemic? Ann Oncol 2010;21(4):680.

24. Farmer, Frenk, Knaul, et al., op. cit.

25. Population Reference Bureau, Alliance for Cervical Cancer Prevention. Preventing cervical cancer worldwide. 2005 [cited 2016 Aug 3]. Available from: http://www.rho.org/files/PRB_ACCP_PreventCervCancer.pdf.

26. Farmer, Frenk, Knaul, et al., op. cit.

27. Central Bureau of Health Intelligence, Directorate General of Health Services, Ministry of Health and Family Welfare. New Delhi: Nirman Bhavan National Health Profile 2016 [cited 2016 Nov 15]. Available from: http://www.cbhidghs.nic.in/E-Book%20HTML-2016/index.html.

28. International Agency for Research on Cancer, op. cit.

29. Byakodi R, Byakodi S, Hiremath S, et al. Oral cancer in India: an epidemiologic and clinical review. J Community Health 2012;37(2):316–9.

30. Pati S, Hussain MA, Chauhan AS, et al. Patient navigation pathway and barriers to treatment seeking in cancer in India: a qualitative inquiry. Cancer Epidemiol 2013;37(6):973–8.

31. Isaac R, Finkel M, Olver I, et al. Translating evidence into practice in low resource settings: cervical cancer screening tests are only part of the solution in rural India. Asian Pac J Cancer Prev 2012;13(8):4169–72.

32. Holeman, Evans, Kane, et al., op. cit.

33. Whittaker R, McRobbie H, Bullen C, et al. Mobile phone-based interventions for smoking cessation. Cochrane Database Syst Rev 2012;Nov 14;11:CD006611. doi: 10.1002/14651858.CD006611.pub3.

34. Ghorai K, Akter S, Khatun F, and Ray P. mHealth for smoking cessation programs: a systematic review. J Personalized Med 2014;4(3):412–23.

35. Cole-Lewis H, Kershaw T. Text messaging as a tool for behavior change in disease prevention and management. Epidemiol Rev 2010;32(1):56–69.

36. Gurman TA, Rubin SE, Roess AA. Effectiveness of mHealth behavior change communication interventions in developing countries: a systematic review of the literature. J Health Commun 2012;17(suppl 1):82–104.

37. GSMA. Bridging the gender gap: mobile access and usage in low and middle-income countries. 2015 [cited 2016 Nov 17]. Available from: http://www.gsma.com /mobilefordevelopment/wp-content/uploads/2016/02/Connected-Women-Gender -Gap.pdf.

38. Mahmud, Rodriguez, Nesbit, et al., op. cit.

39. Surka S, Edirippulige S, Steyn K, et al. Evaluating the use of mobile phone technology to enhance cardiovascular disease screening by community health workers. Int J Med Inform 2014;83(9):648–54.

40. GSMA. Sana Mobile Health Platform case study [cited 2016 Nov 17]. Available from: http://www.gsma.com/connectedliving/wp-content/uploads/2012/03/embsana 0911hires.pdf.

41. Guy R, Hocking J, Wand H, et al. How effective are short message service reminders at increasing clinic attendance? A meta-analysis and systematic review. Health Serv Res 2012;47(2):614–32.

42. Gurol-Urganci I, de Jongh T, Vodopivec-Jamsek V, et al. Mobile phone messaging reminders for attendance at healthcare appointments. Cochrane Database Syst Rev 2013 Dec 5;(12):CD007458. doi: 10.1002/14651858.CD007458.pub3.

43. Lester, Ritvo, Mills, et al., op. cit.

44. Rodrigues R, Shet A, Antony J, et al. Supporting adherence to antiretroviral therapy with mobile phone reminders: results from a cohort in South India. PloS One 2012;7(8):e40723.

45. Population Reference Bureau, Alliance for Cervical Cancer Prevention, op. cit.

46. Barrington J, Wereko-Brobby O, Ward P, et al. SMS for Life: a pilot project to improve anti-malarial drug supply management in rural Tanzania using standard technology. Malaria J 2010;9(1):1. doi: 10.1186/1475-2875-9-298.

47. Githinji S, Kigen S, Memusi D, et al. Reducing stock-outs of life saving malaria commodities using mobile phone text-messaging: SMS for Life study in Kenya. PLoS One 2013;8(1):e54066.

48. Asiimwe C, Gelvin D, Lee E, et al. Use of an innovative, affordable, and open-

source short message service-based tool to monitor malaria in remote areas of Uganda. Am J Trop Med Hyg 2011;85(1):26–33.

49. Zurovac D, Sudoi RK, Akhwale WS, et al. The effect of mobile phone text-message reminders on Kenyan health workers' adherence to malaria treatment guidelines: a cluster randomised trial. Lancet 2011;378(9793):795–803.

50. DeRenzi B, Findlater L, Payne J, et al. Improving community health worker performance through automated SMS. In: Proceedings of the fifth international conference on information and communication technologies and development, ACM, Atlanta, GA; 2012:25–34.

51. Grant L, Brown J, Leng M, et al. Palliative care making a difference in rural Uganda, Kenya and Malawi: three rapid evaluation field studies. BMC Palliat Care 2011;10:8. doi: 10.1186/1472-684X-10-8.

52. Brown T, Wyatt J. Design thinking for social innovation. Stanford Soc Innov Rev 2010;8:30–35.

53. Bannon L. Reimagining HCI: toward a more human-centered perspective. Interactions 2011;18(4):50–57.

54. Kling R, Star SL. Human centered systems in the perspective of organizational and social informatics. Comput Soc 1998;28(1):22–29.

55. Pagliari C. Design and evaluation in eHealth: challenges and implications for an interdisciplinary field. J Med Internet Res 2007;9(2):e15.

56. Brown, Wyatt, op. cit.

57. IDEO. The field guide to human-centered design 2015 [cited 2016 Nov 17]. Available from: http://www.designkit.org/resources/1.

58. Holeman, Evans, Kane, et al., op. cit.

59. IDEO, op. cit.

60. Bannon, op. cit.

61. Friedman B, Kahn PH, Borning A, et al. Value sensitive design and information systems. In: Doorn N, Schuurbiers D, van de Poel I, Gorman ME, editors. Early engagement and new technologies: opening up the Laboratory. Springer Netherlands; 2013. p. 55–95.

62. Miller J, Knott VE, Wilson C, Roder D. A review of community engagement in cancer control studies among Indigenous people of Australia, New Zealand, Canada and the USA. Eur J Cancer Care 2012;21(3):283–95.

63. Thompson VLS, Drake B, James AS, et al. A community coalition to address cancer disparities: transitions, successes and challenges. J Cancer Educ 2015;30(4):616–22.

64. Waller A, Franklin V, Pagliari C, Greene S. Participatory design of a text message scheduling system to support young people with diabetes. Health Inform J 2006;12(4): 304–18.

65. Waugaman A. Implementing the principles for digital development: the principles for digital development working group. 2016 [cited 2016 Nov 15]. Available from: http://digitalprinciples.org/wp-content/uploads/2016/03/From_Principle_to_Practice_v5.pdf.

66. Tomlinson M, Rotheram-Borus MJ, Swartz L, Tsai AC. Scaling up mHealth: where is the evidence? PLoS Med 2013;10(2):e1001382.

67. Lemaire J. Scaling up mobile health: Elements necessary for the successful scale up of mHealth in developing countries. Geneva: Advanced Development for Africa; 2011.

68. Ibid.

69. Tomlinson, Rotheram-Borus, Swartz, Tsai, et al., op. cit.

70. Lemaire,. op. cit.

71. Tomlinson, Rotheram-Borus, Swartz, Tsai, et al., op. cit.

72. Chetley A, Davies J, Trude B, et al. Improving health connecting people: the role of ICTs in the health sector of developing countries. 2006 [cited 2016 Nov 15]. Available from: https://www.infodev.org/infodev-files/resource/InfodevDocuments_84.pdf.

73. Tomlinson, Rotheram-Borus, Swartz, Tsai, et al., op. cit.

74. Lemaire, op. cit.

75. Mechael P, Batavia H, Kaonga N, et al. Barriers and gaps affecting mHealth in low and middle income countries: policy white paper. Columbia University, Earth Institute, Center for Global Health and Economic Development (CGHED); 2010 [cited 2016 Nov 15]. Available from: http://www.globalproblems-globalsolutions-files.org/pdfs/mHealth_Barriers_White_Paper.pdf.

76. Chetley, Davies, Trude, et al., op. cit.

77. Mechael, Batavia, Kaonga, et al., op. cit.

78. Labrique, Vasudevan, Kochi, et al., op. cit.

79. Holeman, Evans, Kane, op. cit.

80. CanTreat, International, op. cit.

81. Holeman, Evans, Kane, op. cit.

82. Mechael, Batavia, Kaonga, op. cit.

83. Qiang CZ, Yamamichi M, Hausman V, et al. Mobile applications for the health sector. Washington DC: World Bank; 2011 [cited 2016 Nov 15]. Available from: http://siteresources.worldbank.org/INFORMATIONANDCOMMUNICATIONAND TECHNOLOGIES/Resources/mHealth_report.pdf.

84. Tomlinson, Rotheram-Borus, Swartz, Tsai, et al., op. cit.

85. Estrin D, Sim I. Open mHealth architecture: an engine for health care innovation. Sci 2010;330(6005):759–60.

86. Tomlinson, Rotheram-Borus, Swartz, Tsai, et al., op. cit.

87. Labrique, Vasudevan, Kochi, et al., op. cit.

88. Qiang, Yamamichi, Hausman, et al., op. cit.

89. Tomlinson, Rotheram-Borus, Swartz, Tsai, et al., op. cit.

90. Lemaire, op. cit.

91. Holeman, Evans, Kane, op. cit.

92. Lemaire, op. cit.

Chapter 10

Liz Grant

The Case for the Integration of Palliative Care in Health Care Systems

Muka's Story

The journey starts on a steep dirt road. It is cold, for we are on the slopes of Mount Kenya, and it is July, the cold month. After passing the last village, the road narrows and turns steeply to pass along the top of a gorge. One side has the spectacular drop into a valley 200 feet below. A tiny path takes us toward a compound. Leaving the car, we walk the last short distance into the compound. An elderly looking man, though he may only be in his early fifties, is sitting outside a hut weaving a basket with the stems he has gathered from a forest vine. It is an intricate task, taking quite a few hours' work for the equivalent of a few cents. He greets us warmly, and we are given permission to enter the hut of his wife, Muka. He returns to his seat beside the kitchen: a hut with three stones, a fire, and two pots.

Beside the kitchen there is a pen for the cow, the family's only steady source of income. The husband carries milk to the dairy every day and uses the money (only a few dollars) to buy the food for the day. There is a small farm next to the hut, little more than a field, with a neglected coffee tree and some maize, beans, and bananas growing there. Water is carried from a nearby stream. There is no electricity.

We enter a dark room that feels cold. It is not until our eyes adjust that we can see Muka lying on her bed (a stained, thin foam mattress) covered with one thin blanket. The wooden slats of the hut do not join evenly, and one has been removed to let more light in. There are some chickens scraping on the earthen floor under the bed, and a line hangs across the room with a few clothes on it. Muka greets us, pleased even in the midst of her pain to have company.

Muka, a fifty-seven-year old woman, is the second wife of a subsistence farmer. She was diagnosed two years ago as having inoperable carcinoma of the vulva. Known by her community as a hard-working woman, she continued working on her husbands' small farm as well as picking tea leaves on neighboring farms until her pain became unbearable. She has borne many children, but only a fourteen-year old son with learning disabilities and a ten-year old daughter who attends the local primary school live with her.

Muka knows that she has cancer and that she is dying. She confides in us that she is waiting daily to be relieved of the pain and go to heaven. I ask if she is in pain. "Not so much today," she says. "I am able to talk. When the pain is too much, I cannot talk." She begins to talk of the past. She wishes she had gone to the hospital earlier; she went "when the pimple was too advanced." She tried small remedies from cheap, private little clinics. When she finally saw a doctor, she was told that the cancer was too advanced. She had an ultrasound examination and believed that the strange machine had made the cancer worse. She was sent home from the hospital with some morphine, but not enough to last more than a few days. She has no money to purchase more. We examine her and find an infected bedsore, which she never mentioned to us.

Muka accepts life as it is. All she can do now is wait until her God calls her home. Her family members know she is dying. She speaks freely about death. Her husband now has to take care of her and the two younger children. Her older married daughters visit regularly, but only the oldest can cope with the illness, and even then, this daughter finds it too difficult to wash her. Muka is not scared of death, but speaks of how her family is scared of her dying. We talk with her and her family about how best to care for her and how to look after her wounds. Back at the hospital base, we arrange for some morphine to be delivered to her.

On a second visit we immediately notice that Muka looks gravely ill and is in severe pain. She asks if we could bathe her, which we do. We use a small piece of cloth from one of the blouses hanging on the line. The rag becomes dirty very quickly as we wash her head, neck, shoulders, arms, upper torso, and legs, then finally uncover her lower abdomen to wash the wounded area. Despite the morphine, she screams in pain as we move the blanket away. The wound is as large as a small football; the gaping hole is white and infected. A huge bedsore on her lower back and right hip is also white and raw. The mattress is soaked in urine and feces. For days, nobody has cleaned her.

It is clear to us that Muka cannot remain at home. Her family, though desperately trying to care for her and doing their best, are just not able to manage for her physically or emotionally at home. We begin the difficult task of getting this woman who cannot bend and is in horrific pain out of her small room with its tiny doorway to the car. As we move her, her young, disabled son bangs loudly and angrily on the side of the hut with a stick. He senses that we are taking his mother away. In the car, in pain from the jolting, Muka begins to sing: "Trust in God on the journey.... In His hands you will not be defeated."

Once in hospital, Muka receives morphine, ibuprofen, promethazine, and bisacodyl, and her pain becomes bearable. At home, she had said that she wanted to die in God's time; but in the hospital, she wishes strongly to die. She dies soon after our visit.

Muka coped with her circumstances through faith. She was not blind to what she did not have: she cried in severe pain; she wished for food when hungry; she felt the cold; she was sad when friends did not come inside; and she knew that her physical, emotional, and social/environmental needs were not being met. However, she had spiritual needs, and these were being met. She was certain God was with her. She waited for His time to call her home; she knew in faith that death was not the end; and she prayed and sang. The act of communing with God brought her comfort. She fellowshipped with members of the church and enjoyed their company. Her identity was bound up in her faith in God. Her cosmology was that of moving on a journey, through hard times, traveling where "those ahead of the journey" had passed, until the time when, as the words of the hymn she sang said, "the body will be left and become dust." She lived and died and suffered her illness within this paradigm. Her suffering was severe, but her faith kept her strong until the end.

The Importance of Palliative Care

For many months Muka's death haunted me. Could she have had a "better" death? Could palliative care have eased her suffering and helped her and her family cope with her cancer? This chapter discusses the importance of recognizing palliative care's role as an integral and integrated component of a health care system.

Palliative care is an approach to care, a care delivery service, and a system of care for those living with terminal illnesses. It is complex and needs to be responsive to the different stages of illness as well as its changing nature. Palliative care addresses cultural, social, and spiritual beliefs about illness and death and incorporates a range of health and social services. It aims to address "total pain" and suffering across many dimensions by affirming life and equipping patients with the tools to "live well" and ultimately to "die well." Palliative care should start not at the end point just before death, but rather at the stage when the patient, caregivers, and clinicians recognize and accept that the patient is living with an illness that is life-limiting.

Numerous components constitute palliative care, and these components shift and change in response to patient needs and circumstances. Palliative care recognizes both the linear journey element of living with illness and the potential circular nature of this journey (the lack of certainty about the timing of death).

Universal access to quality palliative care remains a challenge in low- and middle-income countries (LMICs), as needs and demands far outstrip the supply. Weak health systems, resource limitations, and the dual burden of communicable disease and non-communicable disease serve to complicate efforts to provide efficient and effective palliative care in many LMICs. That being said, there is a growing consensus that palliative care must be better integrated into the delivery of health services in order to become a truly integral component of health and social care as well as a marker of quality of life and death.

Over the past decade there has been a shift in attitude toward palliative care, from offering care to people suffering from particular illnesses (such as cancer) in their last days of life to an awareness that access to palliative care is a fundamental human right for all who are living with a life-limiting illness. In 2014 the first global resolution on palliative care, World Health Assembly 67.19, called upon the World Health Organization (WHO) and member states to improve access to palliative care as a core component of health systems, with an emphasis on primary health care and community/ home-based care. Member states requested that WHO develop evidence-based tools on integrating palliative care into national health systems across disease groups and levels of care. The WHO prepared a practical manual on how to plan, implement, and integrate palliative care services into existing health care services. Specifically, the WHO Global Action Plan for the Prevention and Control of Non-communicable Diseases 2013–2020 identified palliative care as a core part of the comprehensive services required for non-communicable diseases. (1) This resolution provided the impetus for investment in palliative care.

While such action is important, there first needs to be an understanding about the ways in which palliative care programs can be integrated into a health care system and the types of palliative care programs that can or should support and enhance such a system. Interpretations of how palliative care can be integrated into the health infrastructure differ among countries based on organizations, economic, and sociocultural norms. The important point is to have a discussion about its value, then decide how to integrate palliative care services into the health care structure.

Key questions need answers. How should we increase palliative care coverage? How should we develop dynamic and flexible responses to the changing morbidity and mortality realities of a place? How can we harness new technologies while respecting cultural traditions? How can we ensure that governments recognize the value of palliative care? How can we disseminate information about palliative care to the community? How can we best provide high-quality end-of-life services to ensure dignity in death?

To ensure palliative care is recognized as an integral component of health and social care, we need curriculum planning and integration at the undergraduate and postgraduate levels for health and social care workers. There is evidence of the impact of developing integrated models of palliative care in achieving individual, health system, and societal change with an impact far beyond the simple acquisition of knowledge and skills. (2)

Looking at innovative ways in which palliative care has been integrated into local communities can help shed light on how to answer these and other similar questions. Following is a discussion of a framework developed from an action-research program, Integrate, led by the University of Edinburgh-Makerere University, Uganda, and the African Palliative Care Association. (3) Partners worked with the ministries of health, national palliative care associations, and twelve hospitals in four countries in East Africa to develop models of how to integrate palliative care into national health systems. Previous work had identified that existing models of palliative care are divided into four domains: specialist level, district hospital level, health center level, and community level. Investing in strengthening programs that extend the linkages among these segregated models into a whole systems approach has been instrumental in improving end-of-life patient care as well as in adding value to the system of health care delivery. (4–6)

The Integrate program uses a four-pillar approach of advocacy, staff development, service redesign, and partnership, which enabled the creation of new ways of delivering health care that have had positive repercussions for the wider health system. This approach provides a template, albeit in microcosm, of how a model can work across illnesses, across workforce cadres, and across other services to deliver holistic, compassionate care.

A common framework emerged from our work (known as the P Framework), which ensured that each of the areas would be supported. (See table 10.1.) Often it is not about setting up new services, but rather about uniting different separate services and systems to become a whole. It is about enabling services to be in the right place at the right time, supported by people with the right skills and the right resources for care. It requires an emphasis not on expensive tools or top end technology, but on seamlessness.

Strengthening the Health Care System

Strengthening the health care system needs to become a priority if palliative care is to be integrated successfully. The Tallinn Charter of 2008 recognized that sustained improvement in health can only come about through strengthened health systems. (7) Doing so, however, usually requires first understanding and dealing with the constraints, challenges, and obstacles that systems face in their efforts to deliver quality care, including but not limited to severe health worker shortages; fragile infrastructures that require updating and upgrading; an often acute lack of essential and supportive health commodities (such as equipment and medicines); shortage of funds; poorly equipped facilities; logistics problems (such as transportation and storage of supplies); and lack of systems in place to track the progress of, monitor, and evaluate services.

If health care systems are to succeed in the long term in providing high-quality care, including palliative care, several issues must be addressed:

We need to understand that referral systems should be built from community to hospital, within hospital wards and departments, and from hospital to community services and health facilities.
We need to recognize the ingrained hierarchical pyramid of the health worker community and its effects on decision making,

Table 10.1. The P Framework

PATIENTS (who receive care and who also give care to others)

A PLAN of action that captures the vision and outlines the way in which the district envisions palliative care.

PRECEPTORSHIP: training pre-service and in-service.

National POLICIES applied at district level that support the vision.

A district-wide referral PATHWAY that joins providers (hospitals, clinics, NGOs, and others) together.

PROTOCOLS to ensure confidence to make right decisions at the right time.

PURPOSEFUL PRESCRIBING: shared documentation, skilled pharmacists, secure systems.

PROCUREMENT SYSTEMS: steady supplies, making drugs consistently available.

PERFORMANCE SYSTEMS: tools that ensure quality and capture change.

PARTNERSHIPS: a network of support.

PASTORAL CARE and SUPPORT.

PRESENCE: physical places where palliative care is seen.

---

communication, and due process. For example, there are rules about who has authority to write in hospital notes (in many places nurses may not be allowed to) or who has the voice to make service suggestions (nurses and clinical officers may have less opportunity than doctors).

We need to recognize that palliative care aims to embed and exemplify a multidisciplinary team approach that takes into account the pyramid structure of health workers but tries to build in communication pathways both horizontally and vertically.

We need to understand that health care teams are usually quite small and consequently reliant on a few individuals. If these individuals leave, are ill, or cannot work for any reason, this can be challenging for the palliative care team.

We need to move away from isolated islands of palliative care provision that is often delivered outside the hospital by nongovernmental organizations and reliant on external donor funding. We have found that sustainable funding models are only possible with integrated care.

We need to recognize that despite their training in therapeutic and drug management, health workers and patients still hold many myths and misconceptions about palliative care. For example, staff and families may fear morphine, viewing it as an addictive drug. Staff may not fully understand the benefits of administering morphine to end-of-life patients.

There should be more discussion about the stigma around death and dying, especially if the perception of the service is solely about caring for those who are dying (in most parts of the world, palliative care services are most commonly associated with death and dying).

We need to build a cross-disciplinary cross-cadre knowledge base and to strengthen communication skills among staff, patients, and family. In the few hospitals where there are palliative services, the frequency of "blind referrals" (when palliative care teams are called to see patients without the patient having been made aware that he or she is being referred to a palliative care unit) is a common problem. This most often happens when ward staff are reluctant to speak about the inevitability of death to a patient and/or family, see death as a failure of their ability to care for the patient, or decide that it is just not their business to speak out.

We need to understand changing needs and context. Many palliative care programs have been established either as a response to the burden of cancer or in reaction to the rapidly expanding HIV pandemic, especially during the 1990s, when no affordable treatments were generally available in most of sub-Saharan Africa, where the need was the greatest. The difficulties that palliative care programs have in widening or shifting their remit provide a snapshot of how difficult it is for a health system to shift or change from what it traditionally does.

We need to recognize that obstacles arise when donors and/or funders, who view their particular area of commitment as the priority area, require programs to continue to deliver care against agreed objectives, even when the circumstances and needs have changed.

These challenges are deeply embedded in the system of care. Raising awareness of the challenges should be viewed as something positive, as it opens the opportunity to initiate changes. Understanding how programs respond to challenges provides insights into new ways of delivering health care.

The University of Edinburgh Experience in Sub-Saharan Africa

The following short discussion focuses on our experience in the delivery of palliative care in sub-Saharan Africa. Depending on local contexts, which are more often than not shaped by grassroots, local needs and local and national restraints and constraints, our palliative care programs are inevitably structured and designed differently. All have tried to construct and deliver their services through a public health perspective with a primary care–focused approach, which aims to create pathways between and across community, social, faith, and clinical services. Each of the programs had a goal to ensure that everyone, regardless of age, gender, diagnosis, race, or faith, received care that addressed his or her specific medical and familial needs.

Specifically, the programs

Established an innovative "shared care" role modality.

Expanded opportunities of channeling the "health capital" abundant in communities. This was best exemplified through the use of volunteers working in concert with the medical and nursing caregivers.

Provided excellent examples of the possibilities and challenges of integration of palliative care within the local health scheme. Such integration is easier if the program establishes a referral pathway, with each party understanding its boundaries and limits. Engagement becomes more difficult if the program has been set up to deliver everything itself, from diagnosis services, to clinical and social care, to home-based care, to a form of inpatient care in which all drugs and resources are secured by and for the program and are not available for others.

Provided examples of monitoring and evaluation within the palliative discipline that can be integrated with other health and social services.

Provided clinical leadership and decision making to all staff within the hospital or district, especially with regard to reducing aggressive treatments, establishing protocols for drug therapy, and designing clinical care management.
Modeled how to become a training site for others.

We found that health workers with a commitment to care of the terminally ill have a very good idea of the additional resources that are needed in the community to increase the capacity and reach of a palliative care program. Often what is needed is not more money or staff (which are, of course, important), but space and time to work with other agencies already present in the community to extend their services in structured ways so as to create more connected pathways between and across different care agencies.

In Conclusion: Lesson Learned

Our experience working with colleagues in Zambia, Rwanda, Uganda, and Kenya has shown us that the added value of palliative care models lies in the strength of the host country's health care system as well as the support of key policy makers, the medical community, and perhaps most important, the local community. The more formalized the referral system and the stronger the partnership between the program health workers and their counterparts in local health facilities, and indeed the degree to which the health facility workers and the program workers share a similar vision, the greater are the chances of success.

Programs that link hospital services directly to services that are part of the local community are more likely to succeed. Those programs that have strong links with community volunteers, caregivers, and home-based palliative care assistants do better than those that do not have these connections. We have found that families of those who have received palliative care are strong advocates for the program. Those local communities in which the residents are aware of the care that their neighbors receive are often more ready to support palliative care.

However, palliative care programs need to recognize that they cannot be all things to all people. Within all health care schemes, but perhaps most acutely within palliative care, there are many blurred edges between hospital and community, especially for rural hospitals, where communities frequently want direct access to hospital services. Every program must be flexible, adapt to the changing needs of the community, and be respectful of the local norms and mores related to death and dying.

By the time Muka's cancer diagnosis was made, it was far too late to alter her prognosis. Screening might have picked up her cancer at an early stage, which probably would have changed the outcome. However, her last few months of life were anything but high quality. While her faith helped her through her ordeal, there is no doubt that she suffered. Her family suffered. Had she received palliative care, things might have been different. Whereas cancer screening is not always possible in many parts of the world, helping people die a "good death" by means of palliative care is indeed not only feasible, but necessary.

References

1. World Health Organization. Planning and implementing palliative care services: a guide for programme managers [cited 2017 Feb 4]. Available from: http://www.who.int/ncds/management/palliative-care/palliative_care_services/en/.

2. Strengthening of palliative care as a component of comprehensive care throughout the life course. 67th World Health Assembly; 2014 [cited 2017 Feb 4]. Available from: http://apps.who.int/medicinedocs/en/d/Js21454ar/.

3. University of Edinburgh, Makerere University Palliative Care Unit, African Palliative Care Association. Final evaluation report for the Integrate Palliative Care Project. London: Tropical Health & Education Trust; 2015 [cited 2017 Feb 4]. Available from: http://www.thet.org/health-partnership-scheme/resources/case-studies/health-partnership-scheme-case-studies/prioritizing-palliative-care-in-africa.

4. Downing J, Grant L, Leng M, Namukwaya E. Understanding models of palliative care delivery in sub-Saharan Africa: learning from programs in Kenya and Malawi. J Pain Symptom Manage 2015;50(3):362–70.

5. Grant L, Brown J, Leng M, et al. Palliative care making a difference in rural Uganda, Kenya and Malawi: three rapid evaluation field studies. BMC Palliat Care 2011;10(1):8.

6. Grant E, Murray S, Grant A, Brown J. A good death in rural Africa? Listening to patients and their families talk about care needs at the end of life. J Palliat Care 2003;19:3159—67.

7. World Health Organization. Implementation of the Tallinn Charter: Final Report. 2015 [cited 2017 Feb 4]. Available from: http://www.euro.who.int/__data/assets/pdf_file/0008/287360/Implementation-of-Tallinn-Charter-Final-Report.pdf?ua=1.

Madelon L. Finkel

Thoughts Going Forward

The case studies presented in the previous chapters illustrate many things. First, one size does not fit all when it comes to cancer screening in LMICs. Each of the screening programs had to be designed to meet the cultural, logistical, economic, and administrative constraints of the host site. What may work well in Honduras may not in India. Second, initiating a screening program is hugely complex, especially in areas where cancer screening is foreign to the local population. Third, gaining the trust and cooperation of the community and local leaders is as important as it is time consuming. Fourth, planning how to follow up with those who test positive and how to encourage these individuals to seek treatment, especially when they do not have overt symptoms, is challenging, to say the least. Yet this issue is one of the most crucial to consider when designing a cancer screening program. Screening for screening's sake is neither helpful nor ethical if there is not a plan in place to provide treatment after the screening.

The authors raise more questions than they have answers for. What should be clear, however, is that designing and implementing cancer screening programs is complex, challenging, and yes, at times frustrating. Many factors—organizational, administrative, financial, social, and cultural—must be addressed before attempting to introduce screening in an area where such action might be viewed as foreign or even threatening, Without first obtaining the full support of the local population, without first providing an intensive educational campaign touting the benefits of and the need for cancer screening, the program will probably fail. As the economist Milton Friedman said, "There's nothing that does so much harm as good intentions."

For those in the developed world, cancer is a disease that must be "fought." President Richard Nixon's signing of the National Cancer Act of 1971 is generally viewed as the beginning of the "war on cancer." This is a rallying cry and implies that no effort must be spared to find a cure for the disease. Forty-six years after President Richard Nixon declared "war" on the disease, cancer remains one of the leading causes of morbidity and mortality in the world, and finding a "cure" is the dream of researchers and politicians as well as the public. In 2016 President Barack Obama announced a $1 billion "moonshot" to cure cancer, putting Vice President Joe Biden (whose son Beau died of brain cancer) in charge of "mission control." Biden said, "What we're trying to do is end up with a quantum leap on the path to a cure."

Of course "cancer" is not one disease, and an individual cancer patient will respond differently to treatment depending on the type of cancer, his or her genetic makeup, and so forth. Treatment options vary depending on stage and grade of the cancer, as well as patient characteristics such as age, other medical conditions, and personal preferences. For many cancers, active surveillance ("watchful waiting") rather than immediate treatment is a reasonable and commonly recommended course of action. This is often done for prostate cancer and ductal carcinoma in situ (DCIS), a noninvasive cancer in which abnormal cells have been found in the lining of the breast milk duct but the atypical cells have not spread outside of the ducts into the surrounding breast tissue.

State-of-the art cancer treatments are neither equitably accessible nor available to all segments of the population, especially in LMICs and in rural areas. The quality of cancer care can significantly affect the likelihood of survival and the quality of life during and after cancer treatment. Yet structural barriers (such as weak health care systems; lack of facilities, physicians, and other care givers; and transportation), financial barriers (including lack of insurance or inability to pay for care), and patient factors (such as attitudes and beliefs about cancer and health literacy) complicate the ability to provide high-quality care. And in some places, natural disasters cause havoc (see chapter 7, which discusses Haiti).

New (and usually expensive) drugs are marketed as a beacon of hope, yet research shows that many of the newer drugs prolong survival in metastatic cancer by no more than a few months. (1) The costs and the benefits of cancer treatment should be assessed, and the patient's input in the decision-making process should be elicited. New is not necessarily "better."

For many cancers, prevention and early detection can be a lifesaver. In the United States, for example, a 20 percent increase in five-year survival rates in adults with solid tumors has been documented. (2) This remarkable feat is attributed to prevention and early detection as well as changes in lifestyle. The decrease in the incidence of lung cancer can be directly attributed to a decrease in tobacco use.

Early detection of cancer by means of screening, however useful, does not lend itself to all cancers. The controversy over mammography as a screening tool for breast cancer continues. (3) Screening for colorectal cancer by colonoscopy is effective but expensive and invasive. There are no sensitive and specific tests for early detection of ovarian cancer. And so forth. However, early detection and screening of cervical and oral cancers do make a difference and meet the criteria for screening tests laid out in chapter 2.

Cervical and oral cancers in particular have a high prevalence; if detected at an early stage, they have a very favorable prognosis. If left untreated, the mortality is high. Fortunately there are inexpensive, low-tech ways to detect precancerous and cancerous cervical and oral lesions that are perfect for addressing the challenges in LMICs. One does not need sophisticated technology to detect these cancers. The benefits far outweigh doing nothing.

The chapters in this book describe the challenges, limitations, and successes of low-tech cancer screening. While each example had a slightly different approach to screening, the objectives were the same: save lives by early detection and treatment. Unfortunately, in many of the programs described herein, there is a serious problem of follow-up with those who test positive. In most cases the individual will not go for further testing or treatment because he or she is feeling fine and is symptom free. In other cases the individual is afraid to go for treatment or cannot afford it. In yet other instances, a husband may refuse to allow his wife to seek necessary care. There is nothing more heartbreaking than knowing that early treatment can make a huge difference (in many cases a lifesaving difference), yet failing to convince an individual to come back for care. Every author spoke of this predicament, and each made the case for educational programs that must precede a screening program. Using mobile technology to provide educational messages is an excellent way to bridge the gap between lack of knowledge and seeking care, although there are inherent challenges and problems with dissemination of mobile phones and "cellular challenges" (including connectivity problems). The issue of who pays for the mobile technology must also be resolved before embarking on a plan to incorporate mobile technology into a screening program.

Regarding cervical cancer, many of the authors called for the widespread immunization of young girls as a means of protection against cervical cancer in adulthood. The vaccines have been shown to be effective against the major HPV types known to cause cervical cancer. While the long-term benefits of immunization are apparent for preteen sexually inactive females, women who are not immunized will need to be screened and monitored through adulthood.

Changes in habits (such as decreasing use of tobacco and betel quid) would do much to help reduce the incidence of oral cancer. Oral cavity screening is simple and cheap to do and should be routinely performed at local clinics. Once oral cancer is diagnosed, it usually is too late. Surgical excision of lesions is often disfiguring and somewhat ineffective, and the prognosis for late-stage oral cavity cancer is poor.

Despite health care workers' best efforts, people will continue to die of cancer. In most instances, especially in the LMICs, the dying process is prolonged, painful, and short on dignity. Palliative care can do much to ease the suffering of the patient and his or her family. Palliative care aims to relieve suffering in all stages of disease and is not limited to end of life care. Palliative medicine services, including setting patient-centered, achievable goals for medical care and aggressive symptom management, should be routinely offered alongside curative and disease-modifying treatments for patients with serious illnesses. There is no excuse for a terminally ill individual dying in pain.

In conclusion, this book is not meant to be an exhaustive presentation of the benefits of cancer screening. It is intended to present innovative programs as an illustration of what can be done in rural poor areas of the world. It seeks to challenge those working in global public health to think outside the box and to think of what could be done rather than what cannot be.

"Those who say it cannot be done
should not interrupt those doing it."
—Chinese proverb

References

1. Wise PH. Cancer drugs, survival, and ethics. BMJ 2016;355:i5792.

2. Cancer treatment and survivorship facts and figures 2014–2015 [cited 2017 Feb 6]. Available from: https://www.cancer.org/content/dam/cancer-org/research/cancer-facts-and-statistics/cancer-treatment-and-survivorship-facts-and-figures/cancer-treatment-and-survivorship.

3. Mammography: the screening controversy continues [cited 2017 Feb 6]. Available from: http://www.medscape.org/viewarticle/433989.

Shelly Arora, BDS, MDS
Dr. Arora is working as a senior lecturer in oral surgery at Faculty of Dentistry, SEGi University, Selangor, Malaysia. Dr. Arora earned her bachelor of dental surgery from Manipal University, India, and her master's degree in oral pathology and microbiology from Rajiv Gandhi University of Health Sciences, India. She has been a visiting research scholar at New York University College of Dentistry. Her areas of interest include head and neck cancers, especially oral cancer and oral mucosal diseases.

Joseph Bernard, MD
Dr. Bernard is a faculty member at Haiti's top medical school, University of Notre Dame, where he oversees student research projects. He is trained in infectious disease and oncology and runs the Women's Cancer Center for Innovating Health International in Port-au-Prince, Haiti. He has presented his research at conferences in the United States and Europe.

Shreya Bhatt, MIA
Ms. Bhatt is director of special projects for Asia at Medic Mobile, a nonprofit organization that builds mobile and web tools to improve the delivery of health care in low-resource settings around the world. She has designed and implemented a wide range of mobile health projects to improve health outcomes in areas such as cancer care, mental health, and maternal health. Ms. Bhatt holds a bachelor of science in finance and management from New York University and a master of international affairs in economic and political development from Columbia University.

Christine Campbell, PhD
Dr. Campbell holds the rank of reader at the University of Edinburgh, where she is also program leader in the Usher Institute of Population Health Sciences and Informatics. She is also a member of the Global Health Academy at the University of Edinburgh. Her research focuses on primary care as well as early cancer diagnosis, including her research on cervical cancer screening in Malawi.

Heather A. Cubie, MBE, BSc, MSc, PhD, FRCPath, FRSE
Dr. Cubie is a consultant clinical scientist in virology and founder director of the National HPV Reference Laboratory, based in the Royal Infirmary of Edinburgh. She was head of the HPV Research Group, University of Edinburgh until July 2014 and

184 | About the Contributors

created the Scottish HPV Archive and Scottish HPV Investigators' Network (SHINe). She holds an honorary chair at the University of Edinburgh, is currently a senior adviser to the Global Health Academy, and is responsible for establishing a cervical cancer reduction program in Central Malawi.

Vincent DeGennaro Jr., MD, MPH

Dr. DeGennaro is assistant professor, Division of Hospital Medicine and Division of Global Medicine and Infectious Disease, University of Florida College of Medicine, and affiliate faculty, Center for Latin American Studies, University of Florida. He is president of Innovating Health International, which is based in Haiti. He has years of experience working in developing countries, including Rwanda, where he helped build a national cancer treatment program and a pathology laboratory, and Haiti, where he established a chemotherapy program and a pathology laboratory in Cap Haitien. His research interests include genome sequencing of breast cancer and chronic disease management using point-of-care blood tests, community health workers, and awareness programs.

Jay Evans, MS

Mr. Evans is the regional director for Asia at Medic Mobile and is currently based in Nepal. He is also a lecturer at the University of Edinburgh, Global Health Academy, and adviser to the eHealth Program. He has worked in international development in Asia, Europe, and Latin America in the fields of public health and housing. Jay's team has managed dozens of public health and development projects around the globe in countries such as Mexico, Brazil, Honduras, India, Bangladesh, Egypt, Singapore, Russia, and Costa Rica.

Madelon L. Finkel, PhD

Dr. Finkel is professor of health care policy and research (formerly professor of public health) at Weill Cornell Medical College and was appointed the medical school's first director of the Office of Global Health Medical Education. Her background is in epidemiology and health policy, with a focus on women's health issues. She has conducted seminal research on unconventional gas development and its impact on health. She has served as consultant to numerous law firms, pharmaceutical companies, and health care organizations on matters pertaining to epidemiology. She serves as secretary of the board of the Christian Medical College, Vellore Foundation (USA), and secretary of the board for PSE Healthy Energy, a research and policy nonprofit organization focused on energy policy. She is the author of more than one hundred articles and thirteen books.

Liz Grant, PhD, MFPH, FRCPE

Dr. Grant is the director of the Global Health Academy and assistant principal for Global Health at the University of Edinburgh. She holds the rank of senior lecturer in Global Health and Development in the Usher Institute at the University of Edinburgh and codirects the online master in family medicine, the MSc in global health non-communicable diseases, and the MSc in global eHealth. Dr. Grant also leads the international palliative care and spiritual and palliative care strands within the Primary Palliative Care Research Group in the Centre for Population Health Sciences.

Rita Isaac, MD, MPH

Dr. Isaac is professor of community medicine and head of the RUHSA (Rural Unit for Health and Social Affairs) Department, Christian Medical College, Vellore, India. Since 2007 she has been working on an innovative, feasible model of the "Educate, Screen, Treat" Cervical Cancer preventive program using low-tech methods for rural women in India and more recently, an oral cancer prevention program for rural India. Her other research areas include nutritional issues in adults and children in collaboration with the University of Aberdeen; HIV disease, intestinal dysfunction, and inflammation, supported by the US National Institute of Health; and Empower ASHAs to provide mobile, multiplex, antenatal screening at point of care in collaboration with McGill University, Montreal. She is also currently serving as deputy director (promotion and publicity) at Christian Medical College, Vellore.

Linda S. Kennedy, MEd

Ms. Kennedy is associate director for community affairs at Dartmouth-Hitchcock Medical Center. She is a facilitator and planner who connects people with opportunities and communicates about science to audiences, including the general public, investigators, and poor people who live in low-income countries. For more than twelve years she has been dedicated to community building in a small region of rural Honduras and to developing a research infrastructure there and in urban Honduras. She facilitates research in cancer prevention that yields immediate benefits for local people; improves local care; and makes substantive translational contributions to cancer control with initiatives that are feasible, acceptable, and effective.

A. Ross Kerr, DDS, MSD

Dr. Kerr received his DDS from McGill University and his MSD and certificate in oral medicine at the University of Washington. He is a clinical professor in the Department of Oral and Maxillofacial Pathology, Radiology and Medicine at New York University College of Dentistry. He is a diplomate of the American Board of Oral Medicine and past president of the American Academy of Oral Medicine. He is chair of the Global Oral Cancer Forum and a member of the scientific advisory board for the Oral Cancer Foundation. His interests include the early detection of oral cancer and the diagnosis and management of oral, potentially malignant disorders.

Shobha S. Krishnan, MD, FAAFP

Dr. Krishnan is a board-certified family physician and gynecologist. She has been involved in the area of women's health for over thirty years. She is founder and president of Global Initiative Against HPV and Cervical Cancer. Dr. Krishnan is a member of the expert's panel of the American Sexual Health Association, Medical Advisory Board member of the National Cervical Cancer Coalition, and the scientific advisory committee of the Akbaraly Foundation, Madagascar. In addition, she has served on the STD research-working group at the Columbia College of Physicians and Surgeons and as surveillance physician for the Centers for Disease Control and Prevention. Dr. Krishnan is the author of the national and international award-winning book *The HPV Vaccine Controversy: Sex, Cancer, God, and Politics* (Praeger 2008).

Kaitlin McCurdy, MD

Dr. McCurdy is a hospitalist at the University of Florida in Gainesville. She works with the Global Health Fellowship and with Innovating Health International's cancer treatment program through the University of Florida in Port-au-Prince, Haiti.

Biswajit Paul, MBBS, MD, MIAPSM

Dr. Paul graduated from the Sambalpur University, India, in 2001. He worked as medical officer for the Indian Railways, government of India for two years. He was trained in the specialty of community medicine at SCB Medical College, India, where he obtained his MD in 2008. He joined the Christian Medical College, Vellore, in 2013 and is presently working as associate professor in the Rural Unit for Health and Social Affairs (RUHSA). He is involved in patient care, community development projects, teaching, and research. His fields of interest in research are cervical and oral cancer prevention, cardiovascular disease prevention, and poisoning.

Paul M. Speight, BDS, PhD, FDSRCPS, FDSRCS(Eng), FDSRCS(Ed), FRCPath

Dr. Speight is a professor of oral and maxillofacial pathology at the School of Clinical Dentistry, University of Sheffield. He has served on numerous national and international committees, including for IADR, REF2014, NIHR, and Health Education England. He is current chair of the Scottish Dental Academic Board and of the Research and Awards Committees at the Faculty of Dental Surgery, Royal College of Surgeons of England. His research interests include the pathobiology of oral cancer and oral cancer screening. He has led a number of studies evaluating screening tests and has undertaken cost-effectiveness studies of screening programs. He has advised the UK Department of Health on oral cancer screening.

Grace Tillyard

Ms. Tillyard is currently pursuing a doctoral degree in the Media and Communications Department at Goldsmiths College, London, where she is a Stuart Hall Foundation scholar. For the past four years she has worked in women's health and international development in Haiti, London, and Italy. She holds the position of director of outreach and communication for Innovating Health International, a nonprofit based in Port-au-Prince. Her research interests include feminist cultural approaches to science and technology, women's health, and the Internet and media cultures of use.

Gregory J. Tsongalis, PhD, HCLD, CC
Dr. Tsongalis is the director of the Laboratory for Clinical Genomics and Advanced Technology (CGAT) at the Dartmouth-Hitchcock Medical Center and Norris Cotton Cancer Center in Lebanon, New Hampshire, and a professor of pathology at the Geisel School of Medicine at Dartmouth in Hanover, New Hampshire. His area of expertise is clinical molecular diagnostic applications. His research interests include the pathogenesis of human cancers, personalized medicine, and disruptive technologies. He has authored or edited ten textbooks in the field of molecular pathology, has published more than 200 peer-reviewed manuscripts, and has been an invited speaker at both national and international meetings.

David Weller, MBBS, MPH, PhD, FAFPHM, FRACGP, FRCGP, FRCP
Dr. Weller graduated from the University of Adelaide in 1982 and undertook general practice and public health training in the United Kingdom and Australia (including the MPH at University of Adelaide, 1989–1990). After holding senior lecturer posts in Australia, he moved to Edinburgh in 2000, where he is the James Mackenzie Professor of General Practice and codirector of the Centre for Population Health Sciences. He was head of school from 2005 to 2012 and was director for taught master's programs in the medical school from 2013 to 2015. He is currently international dean for East/South East Asia and Australasia. His research is mainly in cancer prevention and management, and he leads the Cancer and Primary Care Research International Network (Ca-PRI). David sits on various Scottish and UK cancer advisory boards and since 2013 has been editor in chief of the *European Journal of Cancer Care*.